Care of the dying:
A pathway to excellence

John Ellershaw

Susie Wilkinson

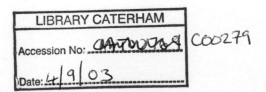
OXFORD
UNIVERSITY PRESS

£24·95

OXFORD

UNIVERSITY PRESS

Great Clarendon Street, Oxford OX2 6DP

Oxford University Press is a department of the University of Oxford.
It furthers the University's objective of excellence in research, scholarship,
and education by publishing worldwide in

Oxford New York

Auckland Bangkok Buenos Aires Cape Town Chennai
Dar es Salaam Delhi Hong Kong Istanbul Karachi Kolkata
Kuala Lumpur Madrid Melbourne Mexico City Mumbai Nairobi
São Paulo Shanghai Taipei Tokyo Toronto

Oxford is a registered trade mark of Oxford University Press
in the UK and in certain other countries

Published in the United States
by Oxford University Press Inc., New York

© Oxford University Press 2003

A catalogue record for this title is available from the British Library

Library of Congress Cataloging in Publication Data
(Data available)
ISBN 0 19 850933 2

10 9 8 7 6 5 4 3 2 1

Typeset by Newgen Imaging Systems (P) Ltd., Chennai, India
Printed in Great Britain
on acid-free paper by
T. J. International Ltd., Padstow

Care of the dying

This book is to be returned on or before
the last date stamped below.

Foreword

Cicely Saunders

"We cannot take away the whole hard thing that is happening, but we can help to bring the burden into manageable proportions." (1)

The above contribution to a seminar on pain in 1962 was an early attempt to present an approach to the 'total pain' that may be faced by a whole family group as one of its members approaches death. Detailed reports of 900 patients in St Joseph's Hospice where the regular giving of opiates was introduced from 1958 had, by the early 1960s shown that neither tolerance nor drug dependence need be clinical problems. It was claimed that the end of life could be a time of achievement for both patients and families, leaving the latter with good memories. That such studies should influence both the introduction of specialist research and education centres and be incorporated into the whole health care system, were aims from the beginning.

The challenges presented by the crisis of imminent death are frequently not recognized and patients and families are parted with little opportunity for dealing with unfinished business or making important farewells. The detailed and much quoted USA Support Study showed how common this was in a number of general hospitals, with poor communication and symptom control remaining unaddressed even after a sustained effort to change this unsatisfactory situation (2).

The introduction of specialist multidisciplinary teams to general hospitals started in the 1970s and since then the spread of palliative care world-wide has often begun with such initiatives. The increasing body of research-based knowledge from the special centres, shared with the ward teams, has shown that the earlier they are involved the easier has been the final course of illness, and that changing gear and simplifying therapy to appropriate levels has been less fraught for both staff and family.

In his book 'Death foretold' Christakis has brought together detailed evidence of the difficulty doctors experience in presenting a poor prognosis. He writes, "the ritualization of optimism, although useful in many respects, can also have negative effects. It may lead physicians and patients to make choices that are ultimately harmful to patients and their families. At its starkest, too much optimism near the end of life may mean patients never see the end coming, never prepare for it, and fight vainly against it." (3)

If the general ward team, initially with information and support from the palliative care team, can demonstrate that the end of life can be effectively eased, it gives comfort and confidence to all concerned. "I just want to go off peaceful, like that old lady over there", said a patient interviewed for a hospice video and, "Efficiency is very comforting", commented a bereaved relative at a day after death meeting.

Much of the now considerable knowledge base has come from the initial concentration on death from cancer but the time has now certainly come for its wider dissemination. "At the outset of a new initiative it is good practice to establish or pilot a project in a single group and a standard process in health service research. Cancer patients were an identifiable group with suffering and pain." (4) Justice certainly demands that people dying from any disease in general hospital wards or in the community should reap the benefits of the early work.

The introduction of care pathways has been an example of collaboration across disciplines and directorates. Preparing the ground for such a pathway for care of the dying is an essential part of this process. Sharing expertise with perceptive leadership helps the varied group involved with any one person's care become a confident team ready to assess the priorities of the new situation. Recognizing that the time has come for this change of gear is then easier as a new and still positive goal is established. Crisis can focus minds and initiate change.

The 'total pain' of the end of life (5) has more components than the physical. Emotional, social, and spiritual needs are detailed in the care pathway. Although the patient may seem semi-conscious at this stage, the way care is given can still reach the most hidden places. The knowledge that the most important person is present or is coming can make a difference even at the end. So many patients slip away just when a family member has left after a long vigil, that it seems there must often be some reason for this. Perhaps it is a subconscious holding back on the part of the relative or a desire on the part of the patient to spare the pain of that last moment of letting go. It may be important for staff to talk about this to assuage hampering guilt. The reported presence of a known member of staff at that moment may heal memories.

Spiritual need includes familiar rituals but goes further than that. While words hallowed by centuries of use can seem of sudden and helpful relevance, a wordless presence may be all that is needed to bring a whole life to a moment of dignity beyond physical loss.

All the careful details of the pathway discussed in this book are a salute to the enduring worth of an individual life. Such an ending can help those left behind to pick up the threads of memory and begin to move forward. That this should be easier to achieve, not only in hospices and their home care outreach, but also in general hospitals, community care, and nursing homes, will be the result of this significant book. Its pragmatic and yet holistic approach has come from the specialist palliative care teams and their research and teaching of the past years. Specialist expertise and general challenge meet here in the dimension of our common humanity.

References

1. **Saunders, C.** (1963). The treatment of intractable pain in terminal cancer. *Proc. R. Soc. Med.,* **56**, 195–7.
2. **The SUPPORT Principal Investigators.** (1995). A controlled trial to improve care for seriously ill hospitalised patients. *J. Am. Med. Assoc.,* **274**, 1591–8.
3. **Christakis, N. A.** (1999). *Death foretold: Prophecy and prognosis in medical care,* p. 178. University of Chicago Press, Chicago and London.
4. **Wasson, K. and George, R.** (2001). Specialist palliative care for non-cancer patients: The ethical arguments. In *Palliative care for non-cancer patients* (ed. J. M. Addington-Hall and I. J. Higginson), pp. 234–43. Oxford University Press, Oxford.
5. **Clark, D.** (1999). Total pain: Disciplinary power and the body in the work of Cicely Saunders 1958–67. *Soc. Sci. Med.,* **49**, 727–36.

Contents

Contributor list

Kim Barrow
Education Facilitator, Marie Curie Centre
Liverpool, Speke Road, Woolton, Liverpool L25
8QA, UK.

Andrew Dickman
Pharmacist, Marie Curie Centre Liverpool,
Speke Road, Woolton, Liverpool L25 8QA, UK.

John Ellershaw
Medical Director, Marie Curie Centre Liverpool,
Speke Road, Woolton, Liverpool L25 8QA, UK.

Alison Foster
Team Leader, Macmillan Palliative Care Team,
Nightingale House Hospice, Chester Road,
Wrexham LL11 2SJ, UK.

Eve Garrard
Department of Philosophy, Keele University,
Keele, Staffordshire, UK.

Paul Glare
Area Director, Palliative Care, Central Sydney
Area Health Service, Royal Prince Alfred
Hospital Road, Missenden Road, Camperdown
NSW 2050, Australia.

Margaret Goodman
Research Assistant, Marie Curie Palliative Care
Research and Development Unit, Department of
Psychiatry, Royal Free & University College
Medical School, University College Medical
School University College London, Royal Free
Campus, Rowland Hill Street, London NW3
2PF, UK.

Margaret Kendall
Nurse Consultant in Palliative Care, Warrington
Hospital, Lovely Lane, Warrington, Cheshire
WA5 1QG, UK.

Carol Kinder
Research Assistant, Marie Curie Centre
Liverpool, Speke Road, Woolton, Liverpool L25
8QA, UK.

Carole Mula
Nurse Consultant Adult Palliative Care, Christie
Hospital, Wilmslow Road, Withington,
Manchester M20 4BX, UK.

Deborah Murphy
Team Leader/Manager, 1st Floor, Linda
McCartney Centre, Royal Liverpool University
Hospitals, Prescot Street, Liverpool L7 8XP, UK.

Sue Overill
Integrated Care Manager, Fourth Floor, Linda
McCartney Centre, Royal Liverpool University
Hospitals, Prescot Street, Liverpool L7 8XP, UK.

Elaine Rosser
Centre Manager, Marie Curie Centre Liverpool,
Speke Road, Woolton, Liverpool L25 8QA, UK.

Cicely Saunders
President, St Christopher's Hospice, 51–59
Lawrie Park Road, London SE26 6DZ, UK.

Peter Speck
Trust Chaplaincy Team Leader, Southampton
University Hosptials NHS Trust, Southampton
General Hospital, Tremona Road, Southampton
SO6 6YD, UK.

Andrew Thorns
Medical Director/Consultant in Palliative
Medicine, Pilgrims Hospice in Thanet,
Ramsgate Road, Margate, Kent CT9 4AD, UK.

Suise Wilkinson
Head of Palliative Care Research, Marie Curie
Palliative Care Research and Development Unit,
Department of Psychiatry, Royal Free &
University College Medical School, University
College Medical School University College
London, Royal Free Campus, Rowland Hill
Street, London NW3 2PF, UK.

Introduction

John Ellershaw

The way we care for the dying reflects to some degree the kind of society that we have created and live in. At the beginning of the 20th Century the majority of deaths in the UK took place in the community. During the 20th Century medicalization and institutionalization of dying patients increased. Today over 66% of patients die in hospital (1).

One of the main forces behind the development of the hospice movement was a reaction against the medical model of disease, diagnosis, and cure (2). It questioned the practice of not telling patients that they had cancer and neglecting incurable or dying patients. Instead the focus was placed on excellence of care for the dying patient. This care included the physical, psychological, social, and spiritual suffering of the patient and those who were important to them.

Palliative care is an approach which improves the quality of life of patients and their families facing the problem associated with life-threatening illness, through the prevention and relief of suffering by means of early identification and impeccable assessment and treatment of pain and other problems, physical, psychosocial, and spiritual. Palliative care:

(a) Provides relief from pain and other distressing symptoms.

(b) Affirms life and regards dying as a normal process.

(c) Intends neither to hasten or postpone death.

(d) Integrates the psychological and spiritual aspects of patient care.

(e) Offers a support system to help patients live as actively as possible until death.

(f) Offers a support system to help the family cope during the patient's illness and in their own bereavement.

(g) Uses a team approach to address the needs of patients and their families, including bereavement counselling, if indicated.

(h) Will enhance quality of life, and may also positively influence the course of illness.

(i) Is applicable early in the course of illness, in conjunction with other therapies that are intended to prolong life, such as chemotherapy or radiation therapy, and includes those investigations needed to better understand and manage distressing clinical complications (3).

During the last half of the 20th Century, the hospice movement developed a model of care that has since been espoused throughout the health care system not only in the UK, but across the world (4, 5). It is well recognized within our society and within the health care system that 'hospice' is synonymous with quality care of the dying.

In a society where over 66% of deaths occur in hospitals, one of the outstanding questions of our time has to be: Why has the model of best practice not been transferred from the hospice to hospital settings, and indeed to community and nursing home settings? There continue to be widely publicized cases of poor care at the end of life (6) and also traumatic experiences of bereaved relatives expressed in the form of complaints. The husband of a cancer patient describes the death of his wife in hospital:

"I lost my wife to cancer of the stomach. She was only 44 when she died. Fifteen minutes before she died, she cried out for me to chop her legs off due to the pain. She passed away in very distressing circumstances, in a great deal of pain. She lost all her dignity."

Too often there is unnecessary suffering at the end of life due lack of appropriate care. There are many reasons for this. One of the main reasons is the fact that palliative care expertise is focused within the hospice. However, increasingly with the development of specialist palliative care teams, expertise has moved into the hospital and community settings. Another reason is lack of palliative care education at both undergraduate and postgraduate level for health care professionals. In addition to this there is a prevailing model of cure which exists within the hospital setting and lack of resources to provide appropriate care at the end of life. This failure to provide good care at the end of life is highlighted in the National Cancer Plan.

"Providing the best possible care of cancer patients remains of paramount importance. Too many patients still experience distressing symptoms, poor nursing care, poor psychological and social support, and inadequate communication from health care professionals during the final stages of an illness. This can have a lasting effect on carers and those close to the patient who often carry the burden of care. The care of all dying patients must improve to the level of the best." (7)

This book will focus on how the philosophy of care for dying patients within the hospice can be transferred to that of an acute hospital setting and how care for the dying can also be optimized in the community and nursing home settings by implementing The Liverpool Integrated Care Pathway for the Dying Patient (LCP). The LCP has evolved and developed over five years. Our experience has led us to believe that it is a tool which can be used not only to influence practice but fundamentally impact on the culture of care of the dying patient in the hospital sector. The LCP provides demonstrable outcomes of care for dying patients and identifies resource and educational needs.

The LCP is a multi-professional document that incorporates evidence-based practice and appropriate guidelines related to care of the dying. The LCP provides a template which describes the process of care which is generally delivered in a clinical situation and incorporates the expected outcome of care delivery. The LCP replaces all other documentation in this phase of care.

A key feature of the LCP is that it empowers generic health care workers to deliver optimal care to dying patients. They can then access appropriate support from specialist palliative care workers. It is often said that doctors and nurses working in acute hospitals do not have enough time to care for dying patients under their care. It is our experience that once health care professionals are empowered to care for the dying, they will prioritize care and endeavour to ensure that patients have a dignified death. The LCP has been developed for care of the dying cancer patients but with minor modifications it has been successfully used in non-cancer patient populations.

The book describes the place of Integrated Care Pathways within the health care system and the introduction of the LCP into the clinical setting including the development of an education programme to support, implement, and sustain its use. It also illustrates how data collected from the LCP can be used to develop standards and outcomes that can demonstrate and influence best practice.

The book includes chapters on symptom control, ethical issues, communication skills, and spiritual care written by experts in the field which underpin the use of the LCP. The book is the result of the experience we have gained during the implementation of the pathway locally in Liverpool, and also by facilitating its implementation in other organizations throughout the UK. We hope that practitioners will find it a useful, practical guide to empower them to care for dying patients to the level of the best.

References

1. ONS Office of National Statistics. (2000). http://www.statistics.gov.uk
2. Clark, D. (2002). Between hope and acceptance: the medicalisation of dying. *Br. Med. J.*, **324**, 905–7.
3. WHO definition of palliative care. (2002) http//www5.who.int/cancer
4. Working party on clinical guidelines in palliative care. (1997). *Changing gear: Guidelines for managing the last days of life: The research evidence* (I. J. Higginson, G. Sen-Gupta, and D. Dunlop). National Council for Hospice and Specialist Palliative Care Services.
5. Twycross, R. and Lichter, I. (1998). The terminal phase. In *Oxford book of palliative medicine* (ed. D. Doyle, G. W. C. Hanks, and N. MacDonald), 2nd edn, Chapter 17. Oxford University Press, Oxford.
6. Dyer, C. (1992). GMC tempers justice with mercy—Cox Case. *Br. Med. J.*, **305**, 1311.
7. Department of Health. (2000). *The NHS cancer plan—A plan for investment, A plan for reform.*

Chapter 1

The development, role, and integration of integrated care pathways in modern day health care

Sue Overill

An Integrated Care Pathway determines locally agreed, multidisciplinary practice based on guidelines and evidence where available, for a specific patient/user group. It forms all or part of the clinical record, documents the care given, and facilitates the evaluation of outcomes for continuous quality improvement (National Pathways Association, 1997) (1).

There are a number of names for the concept of managing patient care through pre-determined, local-based guidelines of care that form the legal record. Those currently developing pathways in health care settings generally accept the definition above as appropriate. In the UK there are many terms currently used. For example, critical care pathways, protocols, and care profiles. This can lead to confusion. Most people seem to refer to the abbreviated 'pathways' as common usage.

Where did care pathways originate

It is generally accepted that the concept developed as a health care initiative in the USA in the 1980s. Originally this model was used in engineering to assess quality in manufacturing by defining processes and auditing variation and outcomes. W. Edwards Deming, one of the principle post-war theorists of the quality improvement movement was influential in getting those involved in delivering care interested in this philosophy and clinicians such as Donald M. Berwick have since established their own international reputations.

Clinicians started redefining care delivery and trying to identify outcomes in a more measurable way. They were focusing on the patient rather than the system and needed to demonstrate efficient progress in order to use costly resources to the full.

Karen Zander was a nurse educator at the New England Centre for Medicine in Boston, Massachusetts in the early 1980s and is credited with developing an approach that she called Care Maps (2) (multidisciplinary action plans). It was felt that nurses, as the profession providing hands on care around the clock, could manage the patient's experience in a more dynamic manner if they had clear indicators with which to measure the patient's progress. The aim was to get consensus from the team on what constituted the significant elements of patient care for a condition or procedure and to maintain the patient's progress. Developing the pathways required collaboration of multidisciplinary teams in a way that was not accepted practice at this time. It also fostered the culture of integrating evidence-based practice and presenting it in a paper format which clinicians could use in their daily delivery of patient care. Benefits were highlighted as staff had greater understanding of each others roles across a service. The use of the pathway resulted in examination of current information given to patients and reviewing these to reflect a holistic approach. When delivering care to their own agreed standard the teams would note variations to these aims. The appraisal of the variations would then prompt discussion and development of critical thinking skills. The ability to collect data on patient outcomes was an attractive incentive to use the pathway for clinicians (3). Modifying the Care Map would facilitate continuous quality improvement and reduce undesirable variations in practice.

This was to be later challenged in the American health care system by process re-engineering and the constant incentive from insurance companies to drive down costs in order to be comparative. However, the concept has stood the test of time and today it is recognized that costs have been managed to the limit and that demonstrating consistent quality of care offered by the individual plans attracts and retains payers, such as Blue Cross. Care pathways can demonstrate how that care is planned and can be appraised by the large insurance organizations. Interestingly, medical insurance companies are known to offer significant reductions in annual premiums to medical staff if they agree to use care pathways as a structure to deliver care. Their rationale is that planned care as set out in the pathways reduces risk and complaint. This is endorsed in the UK as a tool to minimize risk by informing patients of their choices and improving the quality of care (4).

In the UK we have always approached the care pathway concept from a quality perspective with a desire to be effective and efficient with resources but not from the punitive financial approach evident in the USA. Many NHS organizations picked up on the concept and started to develop their own pathways. At first benefits were anecdotal but there is increasing research being done to demonstrate change in outcomes, change management and patient experience. At Central Middlesex Hospital significant work was done in reducing length of stay for orthopaedic patients but innovative practice resulted in this flowing into a hospital at home scheme in partnership with primary care. The organizing of the patient experience into a paper format which staff could read and discuss with the patient was of great educational benefit. Emphasis was placed on the patient and the existing systems challenged with the focus on multi-skilling in appropriate care settings (5).

What is the place of the care pathway in today's health care system

The Government's White Paper 'A first class service—Quality in the new NHS' (6) defined a strategy to support continuous improvement in the delivery of health care.

There were three significant elements within the paper: Clinical Governance, the National Institute for Clinical Excellence (NICE), and the Commission for Health Improvement (CHI) that described a framework for a systematic approach to improve patient care. The initiatives combine an expectation that NHS staff will evaluate care, follow guidelines, and be inspected to ensure compliance. This was the signal to all health care professionals that they must audit the quality of care they delivered and ensure that they evaluate, benchmark, and look for continuous improvement. Earlier the Information for Health strategy (7) had been published which set out levels of progress in working toward an electronic patient record, with time-scales. At level three, together with prescribing and ordering systems online, was electronic integrated care pathways. To those of us who had been developing care pathways this was a direct endorsement of the concept and philosophy that we had been working to fulfil. The Calman-Hine report (8) set the scene for the accreditation of cancer services. This has had a profound effect on the structure of services and ensured that patients are cared for by consultants with adequate experience. The monitoring of GP referrals and hospital response times are increasing the pressure to organize services to meet government and patient expectations.

Three further National Service frameworks have since been published by the Department of Health for Coronary Heart Disease, Older People, and Diabetes. These documents set out a structure that lend themselves to pathway development to capture activity and outcomes. All organizations are required to report monthly to the local Health Authority on their performance against National Clinical indicators. They include topics such as re-admission rates; death following surgery, and form part of national benchmarking which is published in the press. Many organizations have reinforced the view that pathways are an excellent tool to put in place to meet these initiatives. The ability to go across boundaries will become evident as Primary Care Trusts are set up and partnerships develop. There is merit in developing a generic pathway profile that sets out the all-inclusive care and becomes a patient pathway at a local care delivery level. This would require national consensus and would reduce 're-inventing the wheel'. The Liverpool Care of the Dying Pathway (LCP) is an example of how this model can be successfully developed and shared. The challenges of integrating systems across services will be met as the electronic record is developed.

All of these new developments have opened up the care pathways debate. Some of the white papers openly state 'pathways of care' but the context and definition is sometimes in conflict. What is clear is the need for a structure or framework to organize and demonstrate the systems and quality of care delivered across the health care spectrum. Care pathways contribute to this agenda in a most important way by giving responsibility to those actually involved in looking after patients.

What are the key reasons for using integrated care pathways

In order to demonstrate this it is perhaps useful to reflect on how we currently deliver care using an acute health care setting as an example.

A patient coming in for an elective procedure may be admitted to one of a number of surgical wards and the following will influence his or her care.

◆ Experience of medical, nursing staff, and therapies staff with knowledge of procedure.

◆ Number of staff on the ward.

◆ Acuity level of other patients.

◆ Surgeon preferences.

◆ Anaesthetists preferences.

◆ Pre-admission assessment.

◆ Patient understanding of intended procedure and impact on life.

◆ Protocols and guidelines in place.

◆ Staff awareness of those protocols, policies, and guidelines.

◆ Locums and agency staff.

◆ Cleanliness of environment.

◆ Nutrition.

◆ Different documentation across wards, each profession having their own set of records.

◆ Cancelled sessions/no beds.

The above list demonstrates the complexity of delivering care in a safe, correct, and informed manner. Any of the above can influence the quality of the care we intend to deliver but the opportunity to fail is increased if some of these elements combine and there is not good guidance for junior staff to follow. The scenario of a ward that is short of experienced staff, relying on agency or locums who are unaware of local practice, a busy operating day with high level acuity and a planned complex procedure can become high risk. What is useful to counterbalance this?

Those who are responsible for their development say that this risk is reduced by the use of care pathways, which they achieve the following:-

◆ Organize the process.

◆ Identify key outcomes and the tasks associated and avoids duplication.

◆ Foster understanding of individual roles, promotes teamwork, improves communication.

◆ Provide reassurance that the local multidisciplinary team had developed this and it reflects current practice.

◆ Provide focus to support the care givers decision making, proactive problem solving.

◆ Prompt discussion and the provision of verbal and written information for patients.

◆ Have the same document format both for clerking in and delivering care across wards.

- Integrate research, policies, and guidelines into the document.
- Facilitate the recording of routines, such as nutrition, IVI care, drain output, in one place for the multidisciplinary team to read.
- Record when the anticipated outcome is not met and the reason why—e.g. whether inappropriate, achieved earlier/later.
- Reduce inappropriate variation in practice. Contributes to multidisciplinary discussion of variation, justification, and professional opinion.

The development of a care pathway across different settings, even within the same organization, promotes understanding of the constraints and working styles in other departments (9). A pathway covering GP referral, ambulance services, A&E, ward, Care of the Elderly, Rehab, Social Services, and Community Care requires collaborative discussion to take place in order to achieve the optimal benefit for the patient. In many instances this may be the first time such agencies have met for this type of discussion even if they work in the same hospital. The change management element is a great attraction to those developing the pathway. They usually know the blocks preventing them from delivering good care and designing the pathway provides them with both an incentive and permission to implement and achieve a change in practice.

There is the professional and organizational need to ensure that care is delivered to the best possible standard and that avoidable variations are audited and discussed. In order to fulfil the requirements of the internal performance reviews and support the Clinical Governance agenda it is necessary to demonstrate good practice and continuous improvement. Care pathways are an essential part of that reporting structure. Enlarge the scenario and include lifetime management of a patients disease such as diabetes or mental health and the need for a structure which will work for the patients benefit across all care deliverers is very clear. Care pathways are not the only solution as to how we progress but they are an intrinsic part of that development.

There are common elements that constitute a care pathway:-

1. **There is a timeline evident.** This will vary as to the setting, i.e. A&E would be within a short time-scale to reflect the acuity of the situation, a stroke pathway may be detailed over the first week and then lengthen to reflect the rehabilitation stages over a number of weeks. However, the timeline may focus on progression such as an infants weight or a creatinine level in renal disease.

2. **There is supportive evidence of practice.** This may reflect a national guideline, research, local expert opinion and consensus, recent audit.

3. **There is an element of multidisciplinary collaboration.** In practice the goal is that all who are involved document any care or decision making in the pathway so that there is a unified record. Pathways should always be ratified locally to gain ownership and collaboration.

4. **Elements of care are identified, usually, within the time-scale.** The pathway identifies the significant steps to progress the patient's recovery or management of condition. These can also be called outcomes and represent what the team considers best practice by incorporating guidelines, research, or expert opinion.

5. **Continuous review of practice.** By auditing the pathway, either by measuring specific outcomes or by variation analysis, there should be an opportunity to review practice and stimulate discussion and change if appropriate. This can have two time elements:

   (a) At the point of care delivery in supporting decision making as to the appropriateness for an individual patient, using critical thinking skills.

   (b) Retrospectively when analysing data from the pathway. This ties in with the clinical governance agenda which dominates clinical practice currently and enforces continuous quality improvement.

6. **It constitutes all or part of the clinical record.** At the present time there are few care settings using electronic records so most pathways are paper based. This will change as development continues with the Electronic Health Record (EHR) and the Electronic Patient Record (EPR). There are difficulties in combining outcomes with paper-based pathways when the patient has significant co-morbidity's and this will be easier with an electronic approach.

7. **The pathway should cross boundaries.** e.g. A&E to ward, or primary to secondary care. A mature pathway recognizes the broader health management of the patient by linking the contacts. Thus a diabetic pathway may focus on avoidance of admission to hospital, patient education, and prompt feedback if an in-patient episode occurs.

8. **Risk and benefit.** More recently there is a focus on documenting discussion with patients. The ability to diminish complaints and error is facilitated by encouraging those using the pathway to respond to certain prompts. There is merit in including discussion on sensitive issues such as insight and understanding of condition particularly with cancer diagnoses. The benefit for the health care team in having access to such information in one document enables them to have a team approach to supporting patients and their carers.

What are the key stages in the development of a care pathway? (9)

Embarking on this sort of development can be fairly daunting for some staff. They will sometimes be in challenging situations and need support in expressing their views. The presence of an ICP facilitator is valuable to ensure fair play and maintain progress. There are a number of critical success factors to ensure successful adoption of applying a care pathway approach to patient care. It is vital that there is clearly identified support from the executive for the project otherwise it will always be an optional arrangement and success will be limited by that. The appointment of a care pathway facilitator is seen as an essential element with IT skills to create the pathways in a consistent clear format which looks professional. In order to audit the variation and outcomes it is important to have support from the audit team.

Choosing a topic

This may be driven by external influences such as a National Service Framework being published and the service being required to identify how we function in a particular aspect of patient care, e.g. chest pain and thrombolysis management. An existing problem may be identified and devising a pathway is seen by the management or the clinical staff as the way to organize and improve care. It is important that there will be a sufficient volume of patients to use the pathway so that it is evaluated properly and not be too ambitious at the start. Choose something that has a clear beginning and end, which will be achievable. It is always easier to develop any new idea with others who are keen so find some enthusiasts and decide what your remit will be. It is essential that all the team participates to ensure success otherwise when you come to implement there may be dissent from those who were not represented.

Identifying current practice and best models of practice

The most common assumption made is that clinical staff know what happens in their area so there is always merit, when starting to develop pathways, in doing a base review. From the facilitator's perspective it informs he/she on the topic and increases credibility with the team. Audit a sample of 20 case notes to identify current processes and use the results to form the basis of your first meeting. It can be helpful to do this with other members of the team.

Do literature searches and find out what current guidelines, protocols, evidence-based practice (EBP), audits exist and are used by the team. Get samples of pathways from other sources to compare and stimulate discussion.

It is important to recruit representatives to the team who have some credibility with their peers. This can be difficult especially if staff have not been given the choice to get involved.

First meeting

Allow one hour for each meeting and stick to it.

Confirm the topic for development and identify which section of the patient episode you are developing. It may be for the complete episode but a successful approach is to develop sections and bolt them together. A good pathway will cross interfaces so the group should reflect that. Some members may write a section and then leave the group, e.g. A&E episode. Confirm that all those needed are represented.

Establish intermediate and final outcomes of care and include current strategies and agendas for Risk Management, Quality, and Education. Discuss current documentation and integration into the pathway. It is useful to develop a process flow to clarify the pathway and get agreement on what really happens to patients.

Second meeting

Produce a draft and try to circulate for comments prior to the meeting. Confirm that the processes and interactions are correct and that the outcomes identified are going to provide the right information to the team. Start to talk about how staff will be taught about the pathway and who will be responsible. Identify what patient information currently exists and what needs to be written and who will be responsible. Protocols and guidelines may also need to be written. (This can take place in subgroups and brought back to the team for approval.)

Guidelines/protocols may be embedded in the following ways:

1. Inserted as prompts within the pathway.
2. Attached at the back of the ICP.
3. Made reference to in the pathway.

Third meeting

Discuss the second draft and agree changes. Discuss implementation/education needs and time-scale. Are you piloting or implementing across the service? Will you review after a period of time or given number of patients?

Following these you may need more meetings, especially if you have to work hard changing views, encouraging participation, or the topic is more complex than you thought. The ICP facilitator can make sure that difficult issues are discussed and that consensus is achieved. There must be an identifiable benefit for those participating to do this work and if staff feel they have a perfectly good system in place being forced to develop a pathway will require open discussion (10). The base review can be very useful and have significant impact on challenging clinicians perception of what they achieve and how they practice. Many organizations include patients in pathway development and report it as an effective method of challenging professional views.

Education

The team must decide who will target which group of staff to explain and promote the pathway. Use as many people from the design team as possible because of clinical credibility and it is useful to accompany the pathway with a 'how to use' instruction sheet. Include on this a list of the team who developed the pathway so that the users understand that this is a united effort from their colleagues. It can be difficult to capture staff for education and you may find it is better to train some key people on a ward and have them work alongside staff and explain the pathway in practice. All those involved in pathway development agree that education is challenging and time-consuming. However, as you implement more pathways it becomes easier as you are not teaching the principles for the first time.

Patient information is sometimes written separately in lay terms and called a patient pathway. This is given to the patient or carer when the patient commences the pathway and explains the anticipated care. In practice these have been seen as popular with patients and a useful education tool.

Implementation and review

The team should have reached agreement on this topic in the early stages of the development. It is worth clarifying exactly what the remit of the team will be, how long the pilot will run, and how the data will be collected. It is useful to use existing forums to inform clinical staff of the implementation and the purpose and aims of the pathway. Many organizations find it difficult to collect data and implement the pathway with the aim of improving and standardizing practice. Without audit though, the potential for improving patient care cannot be maximized. If systems are in place then the outcomes and variance analysis will be collected and the results fed back to the team. It is important to maintain the group for the review of data as it follows on that improvements and practice changes may need to be agreed. It is important not to have too many trivial changes so that the staff can keep up to date with the different versions but obviously any risk must be minimized.

Each copy of the pathway should include a version number and review date. Each page should have a space to put the date and patient identity number. Notes should be made of meetings to document any changes to the pathway with the rationale supporting the change. These could be needed for legal purposes if the patient care was subject to scrutiny.

As the pathway is used any significant variation must be documented in order to audit the process. It is part of the staff education process that they need to understand the purpose of recording this, otherwise non-compliance will result. This data may be collected in a number of ways:

1. For every patient.
2. A sample of a week or a month.
3. For a specific procedure if a generic pathway, e.g. daycase surgery.
4. By variation only, e.g. daycase surgery when the majority of patients will have no problems.

The group must be clear what they want from the information otherwise there is a real danger, as I found in the USA, of 'swimming in data' that was not useful. It is helpful if there is support from the audit team in the Trust and the data can be scanned or input onto a database or spreadsheet for analysis. When the data is analysed the team need to consider dissemination of the information on a wider scale. This links in with the Clinical Governance agenda and has become a significant reason for the increase in popularity of developing pathways. An important role of the pathways facilitator is to recognize the potential to influence care within an organization. Pathways results need to be shared in order that the team receive recognition of their efforts, share good practice if changes have resulted, and identify trends across the organization. It is at this level that the organization can play a dynamic role in interpreting the results and changing processes. With Directorate performance reviews taking place within Trusts annually there is a good opportunity to collate these results and interpret results to achieve better processes of care. Many pathways involve getting patient feedback and this is helpful information to fuel change. The value of having robust variance analysis is that you can also demonstrate how many times things go well for patients and this is an important factor in staff morale.

The potential for palliative care and pathways

The challenge for palliative care teams is that they often receive a patient referral when clinical staff feel they have exhausted all opportunities to improve the patients condition. Lack of education about palliative treatment is still very evident in many organizations and the culture of failure to cure is in evidence even amongst junior doctors who have had a more holistic element to their training. A pathway can not only initiate discussion with clinicians but can provide the opportunity to educate staff in the most basic of skills and expectations of what comprises a good standard of care for terminal patients. The idea that 'terminal' can cover a long period of time and apply to a well patient is a major shift in the perception of clinicians. For too long the care of the dying has been regarded as a complicated area requiring specialist intervention. By collaborating on the essential elements of care in a progressive timeline within a pathway, the palliative care team can successfully educate staff to take charge of their patients in a way which will meet the needs of the patient and enable them to achieve fulfilment in their professional life. This is especially true when the patient is dying in hospital. A care pathway can identify choices and organize the most appropriate care in respect of the patient's wishes. Guidelines for drug treatments mean that symptoms can be controlled by junior doctors who are often dealing with situations out of hours and with little experience. Family/carer needs can be identified and accommodated within the pathway to ensure that staff are aware of what has been discussed and what is understood. This support gives staff the confidence to believe that they are doing their best for the patient. It also ensures that palliative expertise is sought appropriately for complex patients and does not disempower the clinical team. The standards of care for the dying patient can be transferred with minimal alteration across care settings. If the primary/community staff also use the care pathway they have a full understanding of that standard in order to support families and carers wherever the patient may die.

Whatever the future of the health service in the UK, it is certain that pathways will be an important contributing factor to good quality patient care. This is because the care pathway philosophy reflects the endeavours of clinicians to bring together research, evidence, professional judgement, and common sense to provide the very best care for their patients.

References

1. **Riley, K.** (1998). *NPA Newsletter*. Spring: 2.
2. **Zander, K.** (1992). Critical pathways. In *Total quality management: The health care pioneers* (ed. M. M. Melum and M. K. Sinioris). American Hospital Publishing, Inc.
3. **Zander, K.** (1998). Historical development of outcomes-based care delivery. *Crit. Care Nurs. Clin. North Am.*, **10**, 1–11.
4. **Wilson, J.** (1997). Integrated care management. *Nurs. Manage.*, **4**, 18–9.
5. **Morgan, G.** (1993). The implications of patient focused care. *Nurs. Stand.*, **7**, 37–9.
6. **Department of Health.** (1998). *A first class service—Quality in the NHS*. HMSO.
7. **Department of Health.** (1998). *Information for health: An information strategy for the modern NHS*.
8. **Department of Health.** (1995). The Calman–Hine report. *A policy framework for commissioning cancer services in England and Wales*. London HMSO.
9. **Overill, S.** (1998). A practical guide to care pathways. *J. Integrated Care*, **2**, 93–8.
10. **Claridge, T., Parker, D., and Cook, G.** (In press). The attitudes of health care professionals towards Integrated Care Pathways (ICPs) in Stockport NHS Trust: An investigation' Research project. *J. Qual. Healthcare*.

Chapter 2

How to use the Liverpool Care Pathway for the Dying Patient?

Carol Kinder and John Ellershaw

Why was the Liverpool Integrated Care Pathway for the Dying Patient (LCP) developed?

Over recent years there has been an increasing development of specialist palliative care teams in the community and more recently in the hospital setting. There are over 275 hospital support teams and nurses established throughout the UK. It is unrealistic to expect specialist palliative care teams to be involved with every dying patient. For example, at the Royal Liverpool University Hospital there are approximately 800 referrals to the hospital palliative care team each year. Of these referrals, 70% are discharged home and 30% die in the hospital. A review of the deaths in the hospitals reveals that there are 2,000 each year. Therefore, on average, the palliative care team have contact with only 15% of the deaths occurring in the hospital.

   The Specialist Palliative Care team based at the Royal Liverpool University Hospital together with staff from the Marie Curie Centre in Liverpool, identified integrated care pathways as a potential tool to improve care of dying patients. A care pathway for the dying patient could empower generic workers in the hospital and community settings to follow best practice and also promote the educational role of specialist palliative care teams. In a specialist palliative care unit, it would facilitate multidisciplinary documentation and enable the unit to clearly identify its outcomes of care. In all sectors, by identifying variances, it could facilitate further educational issues and resource needs.

How was the LCP developed?

A multidisciplinary pathway steering group was formed to consider how best to adopt this new culture of integrated care pathways into the palliative care setting. Often the complexity of the measurement of palliative intervention has thwarted effective outcome measures being developed, and it was felt that the physical, psychological, social, and spiritual aspects of care should be included. The group included specialist palliative care nurses, a consultant in palliative medicine, an integrated care pathway co-ordinator and development officer within the Trust, a representative from the pastoral care team, a pharmacist, and members of the ward team.

The steering group identified key outcomes/goals by review of the literature, patient documentation, and multidisciplinary discussion. Further consultation and development was undertaken following discussion with the community palliative care nurse and hospice specialists. Key areas that were identified for inclusion in the document regarding care of the dying patient were:

◆ Identifying patients who were to be included in the pathway.

◆ Initial assessment and care.

◆ Ongoing assessment.

◆ Care of the relatives after death.

The ICP highlights the need to deliver holistic care during the dying phase and gives guidance on the different aspect of care required. It particularly recognizes the areas of care which present most difficulties such as identifying that a patient is entering the dying phase of their illness. The ICP gives the clinical freedom to provide care within an evidence-based framework and acts as a multidisciplinary document which staff can use to co-ordinate and record the care of the patient. The multidisciplinary emphasis ensures that all team members are involved in the decision making process. Key supporting documentation was also identified:

◆ Facilities leaflet.

◆ Symptom control guidelines.

◆ Bereavement leaflet.

What are variances?

If the pathway is not followed at any point, the healthcare professional records a reason for the deviation as a 'variance'. Analysis of this variance provides a mechanism for analysing the reasons for not achieving the desired outcomes of care. This, in turn, directs educational initiatives and resource utilization in order to achieve maximum impact in the provision of clinical care. It is an important part of the care pathway that variances are analysed and acted on when appropriate.

The Liverpool Integrated Care Pathway for the Dying Patient (LCP)

Components of the LCP

1. Initial assessment and care of the dying patient

Cancer patients in the final stages of their illness generally become weaker and spend a greater proportion of time in bed, they are drowsier and less able to take fluids, food, or oral medication. A diagnosis of dying can be made using these criteria and will allow the team caring for the patient to deliver active and appropriate care. A team approach to the diagnosis of dying avoids giving conflicting messages to the family and/or carers. The LCP uses criteria to facilitate this diagnosis. These include when the patient is:

◆ bedbound.

◆ semicomatosed.

+ only able to take sips of fluid.

+ no longer able to take tablets.

It is important to recognize that these criteria cannot always be generalized to non-cancer patients, since the nature of the terminal phase and mode of dying may be different. The LCP identifies that active care of a dying patient should include:

+ Reviewing the medication.

+ Discontinuing non-essential medication.

+ The prescription of prn (as required) medication for pain, nausea/vomiting, and respiratory tract secretions according to guidelines.

It also highlights the need to discuss that the patient is dying with the family and ensure that the religious and spiritual needs of the patient are addressed.

Box 1   Initial assessment and care goals

Comfort Measures:
Goal 1:   Current medication assessed and non-essentials discontinued.
Goal 2:   PRN subcutaneous medication written up according to agreed guidelines.
Goal 3:   Discontinue inappropriate interventions.

Psychological Insight:
Goal 4:   Ability to communicate in English assessed as adequate.
Goal 5:   Insight into condition assessed.

Religious/Spiritual Support
Goal 6:   Religious/spiritual needs assessed with patient/carer.

Communication:
Goal 7:   Identify how family/other are to be informed of patient's impending death.
Goal 8:   Family/other given hospital/hospice facilities leaflet.
Goal 9:   GP practice is aware of patient's condition.

Summary:
Goal 10: Plan of care explained and discussed with patient/family/other.
Goal 11: Family/other express understanding of plan of care.

2. Ongoing care of the dying patient

The LCP emphasizes the importance of regular patient review with at least four hourly observations of symptom control and the need to take appropriate action if there are any problems. Particular attention is given to pain, agitation respiratory secretions, nausea and vomiting, mouth care, bowel care, and micturition problems. There is also emphasis on psychological and spiritual support for the family and patient which is assessed 12 hourly.

Box 2   Ongoing care goals

Comfort Measures

- Patient is pain free.
- Patient is not agitated.
- Patient's breathing is not made difficult by excessive chest secretions.
- Patient does not feel nauseous or vomits.
- Other symptoms (eg dyspnoea).

Treatments/Procedures

- Mouth is moist and clean.
- Micturition difficulties: Patient is comfortable.

Medication

- All medication is given safely and accurately.

Mobility/Pressure area care

- Patient is comfortable and in a safe environment.

Bowel care

- Patient is not agitated or distressed due to constipation or diarrhoea.

Psychological/Insight support

- Patient becomes aware of the situation as appropriate.
- Family/other are prepared for the patient's imminent death with the aim of achieving peace of mind and acceptance.

Religious/Spiritual Support

- Appropriate religious/spiritual support has been given.
- The needs of those attending the patient are accommodated.

3. Care of family and carers after death of the patient

Here the LCP focuses on care and support for the family and carers immediately after death. It includes catering for the information needs of the family and any special request regarding the care of the body.

Box 3   Care after death goals

Goal 12: GP practice contacted regarding patient's death.
Goal 13: Procedures for laying out followed according to agreed policy.
Goal 14: Procedures following death discussed or carried out.
Goal 15: Family/others given information on hospital/hospice procedures.
Goal 16: Hospital/hospice policy followed for patient's valuables and belongings.
Goal 17: Necessary documentation and advice given to the appropriate person.
Goal 18: Bereavement leaflet given.

What does the LCP look like?

The following pages show the LCP on the right-hand side of the page and explanatory notes on the left-hand side, together with cross-references where appropriate to the supporting chapters in the book. This is followed by an example of a completed version of the LCP. The LCP used in this section is the hospital version. The four setting-dependent versions of the LCP, i.e. hospital, hospice, community, and nursing home can be found in Appendix 1–4.

Instructions for use:

1. A method for identifying which patients have been placed on the LCP in your health care setting should be established. This facilitates the co-ordination for analysis.

2. All the goals (outcomes) within the LCP are in **bold** typeface and have tick boxes next to them. Below some goals you will find 'prompts' which support the goals and any interventions you wish to take.

3. If you tick 'NO' for any goal this is a **variance**, which should always be recorded on the back page. It should be highlighted that variances should not be seen as a 'failure in care delivery'; instead they should be viewed as allowing consistency in the care of individual patients.

4. Guidelines for administering pain, agitation, nausea and vomiting, and respiratory tract secretion medication should be attached at the end of the LCP. This offers palliative care guidelines such as converting from MST to diamorphine (Appendix 7).

All personnel completing the care pathway please sign below:

When a patient is placed on a care pathway it replaces all other methods of documentation such as doctors case notes, nurses care plans, etc. Therefore all future written documentation about the patient should be written in the care pathway only.

This section should be completed by any member of staff writing in the LCP as nurses and doctors and including physiotherapists, religious professionals, counsellors, social workers, etc. However, each member of staff need only complete this section once rather than every time they write in the LCP.

Criteria for ICP—Do not put on pathway unless:

The multidisciplinary team (MPT) need to agree that the patient is dying. Generally the patient will have at least 2 of the four criteria identified. (Too often patients die undignified deaths because the health care professionals caring for them have not 'diagnosed dying'.)

It should be noted that if the patient deteriorates when the MPT cannot make the decision such as during the night, it is still possible to place the patient on the LCP. Active interventions can be continued, such as antibiotic therapy until the team make a decision to discontinue them or the patient recovers from the acute episode.

Placing a patient on the LCP does not reduce the level of care given, it can offer a more intense period of caring whilst a difficult decision is being made. If the patients condition improves the LCP can be discontinued it is not a 'one way' pathway.

N.B. The criteria are related to patients with a cancer diagnosis and may need modification for use in non-cancer populations.

The Royal Liverpool University Hospitals – Broadgreen and Liverpool NHS Trust

THE LIVERPOOL INTEGRATED CARE PATHWAY FOR THE TERMINAL/DYING PHASE

A Care Pathway is intended as a guide to treatment and an aid to documenting patient progress. Of course, practitioners are free to exercise their own professional judgement, however any alteration to the practice identified within this ICP must be noted as a variance on the sheet at the back of the pathway.

*Reference: Changing Gear – Guidelines for Managing the Last Days of Life in Adults. National Council for Hospice and Specialist Palliative Care Services. Northamptonshire: Land & Unwin (Data Sciences) Ltd, 1997

CONSULTANT: **NAMED NURSE:**   **WARD:**

INSTRUCTIONS FOR USE

1. All goals are in **heavy** typeface. Interventions, which act as prompts to support the goals, are in normal type.

2. If a goal is not achieved (i.e. variance) then chart on the variance section on the back page.

3. The Palliative Care guidelines are printed on the pages at the end of the pathway. Please make reference as necessary.

4. If you have any problems regarding the Pathway contact the Palliative Care Team.

ALL PERSONNEL COMPLETING THE CARE PATHWAY PLEASE SIGN BELOW

Name (Print)	Full Signature	Initials	Professional Title	Date

CRITERIA FOR ICP – DO NOT PUT ON THE PATHWAY UNLESS

The Multidisciplinary team have agreed the patient is dying and two of the following apply:-

The patient is bedbound	❏	Semi-Comatose	❏
Only able to take sips of fluids	❏	No longer able to take tablets	❏

INITIAL ASSESSMENT

Diagnosis

This should be completed on every patient when starting a patient on the LCP, whether they have a cancer related diagnosis or not.

Physical condition:

This simple list of problems the patient may or may not have is to enable the nurse or doctor completing the LCP an overview of the patient's general condition 'at a glance'. It should be noted that this section is not used in the Hospice version of the LCP, but is very 'popular' in the Hospital version shown.

Comfort measures:

Completing the initial assessment goals/outcomes

All goals, as stated on the guidelines of page 1, have a YES and NO tick box. These need to be completed either by a nurse or a doctor. The interventions under the goals (in normal typeface) are meant as prompts for the nurses to decide whether the goal is achieved (YES) or not achieved (NO/VARIANCE). Again it should be stressed that variances are not a 'failure in care' and allow for individuality within the care pathway. Variances are charted on the variance sheet at the end of the LCP.

For example, Goal 3 states "*discontinue inappropriate interventions*" and lists some interventions below such as blood tests, antibiotics, etc. If we are dealing with a patient who has been placed on the LCP during the night without discussion with the MPT then the nurse can record this goal as a 'NO' and chart the variance on the variance sheet. The reason for variance may state "*antibiotic therapy was not discontinued due to patient deteriorating through the night and on call doctor did not want to discontinue antibiotics, awaiting a review of medical/surgical team*".

Goal 1 (Chapter 3) relates to review of medication and prescribing appropriately for the dying phase.

Goal 2 (Chapter 3) prompts prn (as required) prescribing. Guidelines for symptom control should be attached to each LCP an example is given in Appendix 7.

Goal 3 (Chapter 3, 4) identifies interventions that should be discontinued in the dying phase. It is also important to agree and document that the patient is not for cardiopulmonary resuscitation. If a syringe driver is to be used for subcutaneous medication this should be initiated within 4 hours.

Again it should be noted that in the Hospice LCP the interventions/prompts are removed from under the goals.

Doctors signature:

This section has to be completed by a doctor for legal purposes because as stated earlier the LCP replaces all other forms of documentation. Also if the doctor is recording that the patient is 'Not for CPR' on the lines indicated this signature supports that.

INTEGRATED CARE PATHWAY FOR THE TERMINAL/DYING PHASE

NAME: .... UNIT NO: .... DATE: ....

SECTION 1	PATIENT ASSESSMENT			
DIAGNOSIS	PRIMARY SECONDARY Date of In-patient admission .... Ethnicity			
PHYSICAL CONDITION	Unable to swallow Yes ☐ No ☐ Nausea Yes ☐ No ☐ Vomiting Yes ☐ No ☐ Constipated Yes ☐ No ☐ Confused Yes ☐ No ☐ Agitation Yes ☐ No ☐ Restless Yes ☐ No ☐ Distressed Yes ☐ No ☐		Aware Yes ☐ No ☐ Conscious Yes ☐ No ☐ UTI Problems Yes ☐ No ☐ Catheterised Yes ☐ No ☐ Respiratory Tract Secretions Yes ☐ No ☐ Dyspnoea Yes ☐ No ☐ Pain Yes ☐ No ☐ Other Yes ☐ No ☐	
COMFORT MEASURES	(If 'No' chart as variance on the back page) **Goal 1: Current medication assessed and non essentials discontinued** Yes ☐ No ☐ Appropriate oral drugs converted to subcutaneous route and syringe driver commenced if appropriate Inappropriate medication discontinued			
	Goal 2: PRN subcutaneous medication written up for list below as per Protocol Yes ☐ No ☐ (see blue sheets at back of ICP for guidance) Pain Analgesia Nausea & Vomiting Anti–emetic Agitation Sedative Respiratory Tract Secretions Anticholinergic			
	Goal 3: Discontinue inappropriate interventions Yes ☐ No ☐ Blood Test Antibiotics I.V.'s (fluids/medications) . Not for Cardiopulmonary Resuscitation (Please record below) -- -- Doctor's signature .... Date			
	Goal 3a: Decisions to discontinue inappropriate nursing interventions taken Yes ☐ No ☐ Routine Turning Regime (turn for comfort only) Taking Vital signs **Goal 3b: Syringe driver set up within 4 hours of Doctors order** Yes ☐ No ☐ N/A ☐ Nurse signature .... Date .... Time			

INITIAL ASSESSMENT (continued)

Goal 4 (Chapter 5) highlights the importance of being able to communicate clearly with relatives. In some cases a translator may be needed.

Goal 5 (Chapter 5) does not have an overall tick box for the goal but is broken down into four sections. The nurse must complete all four sections. For example, the nurse should assess whether the patient is a) *'aware of diagnosis'* c) *'has a recognition of dying'* and mark either YES, NO, or COMATOSED, the same should be completed for the family sections b) and d). It is this goal that highlights the need to clearly communicate with the family that the patient is dying.

Goal 6 (Chapter 6) has the overall tick boxes as the goals on page 3. The only difference is that there are other parts that should also be completed. The nurse should tick whether the patient has had a *'formal religion identified'* and state what that religion is, or tick that *'no formal religion was identified'*. If the patient has no formal religion this should not affect the overall goal, this should be recorded as a YES as the goal states *'religious/spiritual needs assessed'*.

Goal 7 If the nurse has *'identified how the family are to be contacted'* this can be recorded as a YES. However, the sections under the goal must be completed.

Goal 8 A facilities leaflet should be given to the family. This should include information on access to the unit including parking, overnight facilities for relatives, and provision of food and drink. An example is given in Appendix 5.

Goal 9 states *'GP practice is aware of patient's condition'*. If the GP admitted the patient to the hospital or hospice because they were dying then the goal can be recorded as a YES. There is some debate whether the GP otherwise needs to be informed if the patient is dying. It is however a time when family members may attend the GP surgery for additional support and therefore it is important that the GP is aware that the patient is dying. It is also important to improve communication between primary and secondary care although it is sometimes difficult to contact the GP practice at night and weekends this should be recorded as a variance.

Goal 10 does not have an overall tick box for the goal but is broken down into three sections. The nurse should tick at least one of the appropriate boxes.

Goal 11 reinforces that the family understand the plan of care.

Both the *nurse* and the *doctor* should sign and date the end of the Initial Assessment section. Furthermore, the person who completed this section should review the goals and all goals recorded as NO should be charted as a variance on the variance sheet at the end of the LCP.

INTEGRATED CARE PATHWAY FOR THE TERMINAL/DYING PHASE

NAME.. UNIT NO: .... DATE: ....

SECTION 1	Patient assessment Contd/
PSYCHOLOGICAL/ INSIGHT	**Goal 4: Ability to communicate in English assessed as adequate** Yes ❑ No ❑ (See Hospital translation policy)

	Goal 5: Insight into condition assessed: Comatosed Yes No
	    Aware of diagnosis a) Patient ❑ ❑ ❑
	                    b) Family/Other ❑ ❑
	
	    Recognition of dying c) Patient ❑ ❑ ❑
	                    d) Family/Other ❑ ❑

RELIGIOUS/ SPIRITUAL SUPPORT	**Goal 6: Religious/spiritual needs assessed with patient/carer** Yes ❑ No ❑ Formal religion identified: .... In-house support Tel/Bleep No: .... Name .... External support Tel/Bleep No: .... Name .... Special needs now, at time of & after death identified:- (please state) ....

COMMUNICATION WITH FAMILY/OTHER	**Goal 7: Identify how family/other are to be informed of patient's impending death** Yes ❑ No ❑
	
	At any time ❑ Not at night-time ❑ Stay overnight at Hospital ❑
	
	Primary Contact Name ....
	Relationship to patient .... Tel no: ....
	Secondary contact ....
	Tel no: ....
	
	Goal 8: Family/other given hospital information on:- Yes ❑ No ❑
	    Concession car parking; Hillsborough accommodation; Dining
	    Room facilities; Payphones; Washrooms & toilet facilities
	    on the ward. Any other relevant information

COMMUNICATION WITH PRIMARY HEALTH CARE TEAM	**Goal 9: G.P. Practice is aware of patient's condition** Yes ❑ No ❑ G.P. Practice to be contacted if unaware patient is dying
SUMMARY	**Goal 10: Plan of care explained & discussed with:-** a) Patient ❑ b) Family ❑ c) Other ❑ d) No ❑
	Goal 11: Family/other express understanding of plan care Yes ❑ No ❑ N/A ❑

If you have charted "No" against any goal so far, please complete variance sheet on the back page before signing below

Signature Health Care Professional   Title   Date

ONGOING ASSESSMENT

Completing the ongoing assessment goals/outcomes (Chapter 3)

This section should be completed four hourly. The goals are again in **bold** typeface and are supported by prompts. The nurse should complete only the goals and record in each column whether the goal was:

- Achieved by recording an **A**.
- Not achieved/variance by recording a **V**.

    For example:

    (a) If the patient is *pain free* at 12 o'clock then the nurse would record an A (achieved) in the appropriate row and column.

    (b) If the patient showed signs of pain or verbalizes that they are in pain then the nurse would record a V (variance). The nurse would then record details of the variance on the variance sheet at the end of the LCP.

The only time the code for **Not appropriate—N/A** is used is for the medication goals. For all other goals only an A for V should be used.

The LCP is completed for each of the goals on this page on a four hourly basis, i.e. 6 times in a twenty four hour period. Each shift nurse should initial the bottom of the page indicating which shift the observations were recorded.

This page is repeated on a twenty four hour basis for the whole time period the patient is on the LCP.

INTEGRATED CARE PATHWAY FOR THE TERMINAL/DYING PHASE

NAME: .... UNIT NO: .... DATE: ....

Codes (Please enter in columns)   A.. Achieved   V.. Variance

SECTION 2	PATIENT PROBLEM/FOCUS	08:00	12:00	16:00	20:00	24:00	04:00
ASSESSMENT PAIN/COMFORT MEASURES							
Pain **Goal: Patient is pain free** ● Verbalised by patient if conscious ● Pain free on movement ● Appears peaceful ● Move only for comfort							
Agitation **Goal: Patient is not agitated** ● Patient does not display signs of delirium, terminal anguish, restlessness (thrashing, plucking, twitching) ● Exclude retention of urine as cause							
Respiratory Tract Secretions **Goal: Patients breathing is not made difficult by excessive secretions**							
Nausea & Vomiting **Goal: Patient does not feel nauseous or vomits** ● Patient verbalises if conscious							
Other symptoms (e.g. dyspnoea) a)							
TREATMENT/PROCEDURES							
Mouth Care **Goal: Mouth is moist and clean.** ● See mouth care policy ● Mouth care to be given at least 4 hourly							
Micturition Difficulties **Goal: Patient is comfortable** ● Urinary catheter if in retention ● Urinary catheter or pads, if general weakness creates incontinence							
MEDICATION (If not appropriate record as N/A)							
Goal: All medication is given safely & accurately. ● If syringe driver in progress check at least 4 hourly ● If medication not required please record as N/A							
Nurse Signature **Repeat this page 24 hrly. Spare copies on Ward**	Early		Late		Night	

ONGOING ASSESSMENT *(continued)*

Completing the ongoing assessment goals/outcomes *(Chapter 3, 4, 5, 6)*

This section should be completed twelve hourly. This page should be completed in the same way as the four hourly section on the previous page.

- achieved by recording an **A**
- not achieved/variance by recording a **V**.

Similarly, it should also be repeated every twenty four hours for the duration of time the patient is on the care LCP.

The nurse again should sign next to the appropriate shift.

The multidisciplinary progress notes section can be used to record any significant event that is not recorded on the pathway. It is not necessary to duplicate information already recorded on the LCP. However significant conversations or specific interventions should be recorded in this section. When the LCP is initiated health care professionals tend to write in great detail in this section. This tends to reduce when people are familiar with the document.

INTEGRATED CARE PATHWAY FOR THE TERMINAL/DYING PHASE

NAME: .... UNIT NO: .... DATE: ....…..............

Complete **12 hourly**		08:00	20:00
MOBILITY/PRESSURE AREA CARE	**Goal: Patient is comfortable and in a safe environment** Patient is moved for comfort only with pressure relieving aids as appropriate e.g. special mattress		
BOWEL CARE	**Goal: Patient is not agitated or distressed due to constipation or diarrhoea**		
PSYCHOLOGICAL/ INSIGHT SUPPORT	**Patient** **Goal: Patient becomes aware of the situation as appropriate** ● Patient is informed of procedures ● Touch, verbal communication is continued **Family/Other** **Goal: Family/Other are prepared for the patient's imminent death with the aim of achieving peace of mind and acceptance** ● Check understanding ● Recognition of patient dying ● Inform of measures taken to maintain patient's comfort ● Explain possibility of physical symptoms e.g. fatigue ● Psychological symptoms such as anxiety/depression ● Social issues such as financial implications		
RELIGIOUS/SPIRITUAL SUPPORT	**Goal: Appropriate religious/spiritual support has been given**		
CARE OF THE FAMILY/OTHERS	**Goal: The needs of those attending the patient are accommodated**		
IF YOU HAVE CHARTERED 'V' AGAINST ANY GOAL SO FAR, PLEASE COMPLETE VARIANCE SHEET AT THE BACK OF THE PATHWAY BEFORE SIGNING BELOW **Repeat this page each 24 hours. Spare sheets on Ward**			

Nurse Signature   Early .... Late .... Night ....…

MULTIDISCIPLINARY PROGRESS NOTES

VERIFICATION OF DEATH

A nurse or doctor can complete this section. The LCP is a legal document and therefore the date, time, and cause of death must be stated.

Care after death:

Completing the ongoing assessment goals/outcomes
This section relates to the care of the 'patient' and the relatives immediately following the patient's death. As with the previous sections each goal must be completed with either a YES or a NO. If No is charted then this is a variance and the details recorded on the variance sheet at the end of the LCP.

Goal 12 it is important to communicate the patient's death to the GP practice.

Goal 13 a procedure should be in place for laying out of the body.

Goal 14 (Chapter 6) if specific procedures or rituals need to be followed they have normally been identified prior to death. It is important to communicate clearly with the family at this time. If a post mortem is required this should be sensitively discussed with the family.

Goal 16 and 17 appropriate procedures should be followed.

Goal 18 (Chapter 5) a bereavement leaflet should be given to the family. This should contain an insight to some of the feelings and reactions that are common in bereavement and contact addresses for bereavement support. An example is given in Appendix 6.

This section must also be signed and dated by the nurse.

Have you completed the last 4 and 12 hourly observations?
This prompt is placed at the end of this section merely as a reminder to nurses to return to the Ongoing Assessment section and ensure they have recorded the patient's final observation. Initial analysis of the LCP found that nearly one third of final observations were missing, however, since adding this prompt to the pathway consecutive yearly data has reduced the missing data around the final observation to approximately 10%.

For example, if the patient died at 2000 hours the nurse caring for the patient will usually be too busy to record the four and twelve hourly observations. The nurse's initial priority will be dealing with relatives and the patient. However, this observation can be retrospectively completed at the completion of the LCP.

Please contact the palliative care team to inform them that this patient was on a pathway:

This prompt is used to inform the palliative care team that the LCP has been completed and can link into the analysis and feedback process.

INTEGRATED CARE PATHWAY FOR THE TERMINAL/DYING PHASE

NAME: .... UNIT NO: .... DATE: ....

VERIFICATION OF DEATH

Date of Death .... Time of Death ....

Persons Present ....

Notes ....

....

Signature .... Time Verified ....

CARE AFTER DEATH	Goal 12: GP Practice contacted re patient's death Date: __/__/__	Yes ☐ No ☐
	Goal 13: Procedures for laying out followed according to hospital policy ● Input patients death on hospital computer	Yes ☐ No ☐
	Goal 14: Procedure following death discussed or carried out N/A ☐ (If yes please indicate) Patient had infectious disease ☐ Patient has religious needs ☐ Post mortem discussed ☐	Yes ☐ No ☐
	Goal 15: Family/other given information on hospital procedures ● Hospital information booklet given to Family/Other about necessary legal tasks ● Relatives/other informed to ring General Office at 10am on next working day to make an appointment to collect death certificate	Yes ☐ No ☐
	Goal 16: Hospital policy followed for patient's valuabes & belongings OUT OF OFFICE HOURS ● Belongings listed and put in A&E Clothing Store ● Vluables listed and put in A&E night safe IN OFFICE HOURS ● Belongings & valuables listed & taken to General Office	Yes ☐ No ☐
	Goal 17: Necessary documentation & advice is given to the appropriate person ● General office booklet given	Yes ☐ No ☐
	Goal 18: Bereavement leaflet given ● 'What to do after death' booklet given (DHSS) if applicable ● Grieving leaflet given	Yes ☐ No ☐

IF YOU HAVE CHARTED "NO" AGAINST ANY GOAL SO FAR, PLEASE COMPLETE VARIANCE SHEET AT THE BACK OF THE PATHWAY BEFORE SIGNING BELOW Nurse Signature .... Date .... *** HAVE YOU COMPLETED THE LAST 4 & 12 HOURLY OBSERVATION**	
PLEASE CONTACT THE PALLIATIVE CARE TEAM TO INFORM THEM THAT THIS PATIENT WAS ON A PATHWAY. EXT 2274	

Variance Analysis sheet:

This is always attached to the back of the LCP.
   When a variance occurs on the pathway:

1. **date of variance is recorded** by the nurse/doctor.
2. **what variance occurred,** such as pain or facilities leaflet not given.
3. **why the variance occurred.** This can usually fall into two types of variance:
   (a) Unavoidable variance, such as pain. This type of variance is unavoidable if the patient is on the correct dose of analgesia and this is being delivered effectively.
   (b) Avoidable variance such as facilities leaflet not given because there was not any available or pain due to analgesics not prescribed. These types of variances would be categorized as avoidable. In both cases prior action should have been taken to ensure that either extra facilities leaflets were ordered/copied or that PRN analgesia was prescribed as soon as the patient was placed on the LCP.
4. **what action was taken is recorded.** For example:
   (a) A facilities leaflet was obtained from another ward and the ward's stock was replenished.
   (b) The doctor was bleeped to prescribe PRN medication.
   (c) The doctor was asked to prescribe a higher dose of analgesic.
5. **nurse/doctor records initials and title**

This process is completed for every recorded variance within the LCP.
   These variances are then analysed and results offer an insight into outcomes of care around dying patients within the health care setting. Furthermore, analysis of goals with frequent variance recordings can identify education and training needs, and resource issues.

INTEGRATED CARE PATHWAY FOR THE TERMINAL/DYING PHASE

NAME: .... UNIT NO: .... DATE: ....

VARIANCE ANALYSIS FOR TERMINAL/DYING PHASE

HOSPITAL

CONSULTANT: ....
DATE OF ADMISSION: ....
DATE OF DEATH: ....
WARD: ....

DATE	WHAT VARIANCE OCCURRED?	WHY DID VARIANCE OCCUR?	ACTION TAKEN	INITIALS	TITLE

An example of a completed Liverpool Care Pathway for the Dying Patient (LCP)

(Hospital Version)

NAME: ......M̲R̲.....S̲m̲i̲t̲h̲......................... UNIT NO: ..1̲2̲3̲.X̲Y̲Z̲....

The Royal Liverpool University Hospitals – Broadgreen and Liverpool NHS Trust

THE LIVERPOOL INTEGRATED CARE PATHWAY FOR THE TERMINAL/DYING PHASE
A Care Pathway is intended as a guide to treatment and an aid to documenting patient progress. Of course, practitioners are free to exercise their own professional judgement, however any alteration to the practice identified within this ICP must be noted as a variance on the sheet at the back of the pathway.
      *Reference: Changing Gear – Guidelines for Managing the Last Days of Life in Adults. National Council for Hospice and Specialist Palliative Care Services. Northamptonshire: Land & Unwin (Data Sciences) Ltd, 1997

CONSULTANT: D̲R̲ A̲   **NAMED NURSE:** J̲.̲ N̲.̲   **WARD:** X̲

INSTRUCTIONS FOR USE

1.   All goals are in **heavy** typeface. Interventions, which act as prompts to support the goals, are in normal type.

2.   If a goal is not achieved (i.e. variance) then chart on the variance section on the back page.

3.   The Palliative Care guidelines are printed on the pages at the end of the pathway. Please make reference as necessary.

4.   If you have any problems regarding the Pathway contact the Palliative Care Team.

ALL PERSONNEL COMPLETING THE CARE PATHWAY PLEASE SIGN BELOW

Name (Print)	Full Signature	Initials	Professional Title	Date
Lynne Jones	L. J.	LJ	Macmillan nurse	01.04.02
L. Chapman	LChp	LJC	SpR	02.04.02
J. Jones	JJones	J.J.	staff nurse	02.04.02
S. Sloan	SSloan	SS	staff nurse	02-04-02

CRITERIA FOR ICP – DO NOT PUT ON THE PATHWAY UNLESS

The Multiprofessional team have agreed the patient is dying and two of the following apply:-

The patient is bedbound ☑   Semi-Comatose ☑

Only able to take sips of fluids ❑   No longer able to take tablets ☑

IF YOU HAVE ANY PROBLEMS

PLEASE

CONTACT THE PALLIATIVE

CARE TEAM

INTEGRATED CARE PATHWAY FOR THE TERMINAL/DYING PHASE

NAME:...mr. Smith.................. UNIT NO: 123 xyz............. DATE: 01. 04. 02.....

SECTION 1	
	PATIENT ASSESSMENT

DIAGNOSIS	PRIMARY SECONDARY Date of In-patient admission 29.03.02 Ethnicity White / British

PHYSICAL CONDITION	Unable to swallow	Yes ☑ No ☐	Aware Yes ☐ No ☑
	Nausea	Yes ☐ No ☑	Conscious Yes ☐ No ☑
	Vomiting	Yes ☐ No ☑	UTI Problems Yes ☐ No ☑
	Constipated	Yes ☑ No ☐	Catheterised Yes ☑ No ☐
	Confused	Yes ☑ No ☐	Respiratory Tract Secretions Yes ☐ No ☑
	Agitation	Yes ☑ No ☐	Dyspnoea Yes ☐ No ☑
	Restless	Yes ☑ No ☐	Pain Yes ☑ No ☐
	Distressed	Yes ☑ No ☐	Other Yes ☐ No ☑

COMFORT MEASUSRES	(If 'No' chart as variance on the back page)
	
	Goal 1: **Current medication assessed and non essentials discontinued** Yes ☑ No ☐
	         Appropriate oral drugs converted to subcutaneous route and syringe
	         driver commenced if appropriate
	         Inappropriate medication discontinued
	
	Goal 2: **PRN subcutaneous medication written up for list below as per Protocol** Yes ☑ No ☐
	         (see blue sheets at back of ICP for guidance)
	         Pain Analgesia
	         Nausea & Vomiting Anti – emetic
	         Agitation Sedative
	         Respiratory Tract Secretions Anticholinergic
	
	Goal 3: **Discontinue inappropriate interventions** Yes ☐ No ☑
	         Blood Test
	         Antibiotics
	         I.V.'s (fluids/medications)
	         Not for Cardiopulmonary Resuscitation (Please record below)
	
	     Not for CPR.
	
	Doctors signature .... Date .02.04.02.........
	
	Goal 3a: **Decisions to discontinue inappropriate nursing interventions taken** Yes ☑ No ☐
	         Routine Turning Regime (turn for comfort only)
	         Taking Vital signs
	
	Goal 3b: **Syringe driver set up within 4 hours of Doctors order** Yes ☐ No ☐ N/A ☑
	
	Nurse signature .... Date 01.04.02.. Time 21.00 hrs

INTEGRATED CARE PATHWAY FOR THE TERMINAL/DYING PHASE

NAME: Mr. Smith   UNIT NO: 123 xyz   DATE: 01·04·02

SECTION 1	Patient assessment Contd/		
PSYCHOLOGICAL/ INSIGHT	**Goal 4: Ability to communicate in English assessed as adequate** (See Hospital translation policy)		Yes ☑ No ☐

Goal 5: Insight into condition assessed

	Comatosed	Yes	No
Aware of diagnosis a) Patient	☑	☐	☐
b) Family/Other		☑	☐
Recognition of dying c) Patient	☑	☐	☐
d) Family/Other		☑	☐

RELIGIOUS/ SPIRITUAL SUPPORT	**Goal 6: Religious/spiritual needs assessed with patient/carer** Yes ☑ No ☐
	Formal religion identified: ...Roman Catholic...
	In-house support Tel/Bleep No: ..123...... Name Father John
	External support Tel/Bleep No: ....Name ....
	Special needs now, at time of & after death Identified:- (please state) ......family requested Sacrament of the sick

COMMUNICATION WITH FAMILY/OTHER	**Goal 7: Identify how family/other are to be informed of patient's impending death** Yes ☑ No ☐
	At any time ☐ Not at night-time ☐ Stay overnight at Hospital ☑
	Primary Contact Name ..Mrs. Smith............................ Relationship to patient ......Wife.............. Tel no: 123. 4567 Secondary contact ..Brian Smith (son)........................ Tel no: 123. 8910..............
	Goal 8: Family/other given hospital information on:- Yes ☑ No ☐ Concession car parking; Hillsborough accommodation; Dining Room facilities; Payphones; Washrooms & toilet facilities on the ward. Any other relevant information

COMMUNICATION WITH PRIMARY HEALTH CARE TEAM	**Goal 9: G.P. Practice is aware of patient's condition** Yes ☐ No ☑ G.P. Practice to be contacted if unaware patient is dying
SUMMARY	**Goal 10: Plan of care explained & discussed with:-** a) Patient ☐ b) Family ☑ c) Other ☐ d) No ☐
	Goal 11: Family/other express understanding of plan care Yes ☑ No ☐ N/A ☐

If you have charted "No" against any goal so far, please complete variance sheet on the back page before signing below

Signature Health Care Professional   L J~~   Title Macmillan nurse Date 01·04·02

INTEGRATED CARE PATHWAY FOR THE TERMINAL/DYING PHASE

NAME: Mr Smith .... UNIT NO: 123 XYZ ...... DATE: 01.04.02 .....

Codes (Please enter in columns) A.. Achieved V.. Variance							

SECTION 2	PATIENT PROBLEM/FOCUS	08:00	12:00	16:00	20:00 21·00 nc	24:00	04:00
ASSESSMENT PAIN/COMFORT MEASURES							
Pain **Goal: Patient is pain free** • Verbalised by patient if conscious • Pain free on movement • Appears peaceful • Move only for comfort					V	A	V
Agitation **Goal: Patient is not agitated** • Patient does not display signs of delirium, terminal anguish, restlessness (thrashing, plucking, twitching) • Exclude retention of urine as cause					V	A	A
Respiratory Tract Secretions **Goal: Patients breathing is not made difficult by excessive secretions**					A	A	A
Nausea & Vomiting **Goal: Patient does not feel nauseous or vomits** • Patient verbalises if conscious					A	A	A
Other symptoms (e.g. dyspnoea) a) ....nil..							
TREATMENT/PROCEDURES							
Mouth Care **Goal: Mouth is moist and clean.** • See mouth care policy • Mouth care to be given at least 4 hourly					A	A	A
Micturition Difficulties **Goal: Patient is comfortable** • Urinary catheter if in retention • Urinary catheter or pads, if general weakness creates incontinence					A	A	A
MEDICATION (If not appropriate record as N/A)							
Goal: All medication is given safely & accurately. • If syringe driver in progress check at least 4 hourly • If medication not required please record as N/A					A	A	A
Nurse Signature Repeat this page 24 hrly. Spare copies on Ward		Early		Late IJ		Night J.J.	

INTEGRATED CARE PATHWAY FOR THE TERMINAL/DYING PHASE

NAME:...*Mr Smith*.................. UNIT NO: ...*123 XY2*......... DATE: *01.04.02*...

Complete 12 hourly			08:00	20:00
MOBILITY/PRESSURE AREA CARE	**Goal: Patient is comfortable and in a safe environment** Patient is moved for comfort only with pressure relieving aids as appropriate e.g. special mattress			A
BOWEL CARE	**Goal: Patient is not agitated or distressed due to constipation or diarrhoea**			A
PSYCHOLOGICAL/ INSIGHT SUPPORT	**Patient** **Goal: Patient becomes aware of the situation as appropriate** • Patient is informed of procedures • Touch, verbal communication is continued			A
	Family/Other **Goal: Family/Other are prepared for the patient's imminent death with the aim of achieving peace of mind and acceptance** • Check understanding • Recognition of patient dying • Inform of measures taken to maintain patient's comfort • Explain possibility of physical symptoms e.g fatigue • Psychological symptoms such as anxiety/depression • Social issues such as financial implications			A
RELIGIOUS/SPIRITUAL SUPPORT	**Goal: Appropriate religious/spiritual support has been given**			A
CARE OF THE FAMILY/OTHERS	**Goal: The needs of those attending the patient are accommodated**			A

IF YOU HAVE CHARTERED 'V' AGAINST ANY GOAL SO FAR, PLEASE COMPLETE VARIANCE SHEET AT THE BACK OF THE PATHWAY BEFORE SIGNING BELOW
Repeat this page each 24 hours. Spare sheets on Ward

Nurse Signature Early .... Late ....*HJ*........................ Night ....*JJ*................

MULTIDISCIPLINARY PROGRESS NOTES

1.4.02   Conducted father John - Sacrament of the sick administered.
          comfort and support offered to family.   HJ.

INTEGRATED CARE PATHWAY FOR THE TERMINAL/DYING PHASE

NAME:...Mr.....Smith.................. UNIT NO: ..123872......... DATE:...02-9A-92

Codes (Please enter in columns) A.. Achieved V.. Variance							

SECTION 2	PATIENT PROBLEM/FOCUS	08:00	12:00	16:00	20:00	24:00	04:00
ASSESSMENT PAIN/COMFORT MEASURES							
Pain **Goal: Patient is pain free** • Verbalised by patient if conscious • Pain free on movement • Appears peaceful • Move only for comfort		V	A	A	A		
Agitation **Goal: Patient is not agitated** • Patient does not display signs of delirium, terminal anguish, restlessness (thrashing, plucking, twitching) • Exclude retention of urine as cause		A	A	A	A		
Respiratory Tract Secretions **Goal: Patients breathing is not made difficult by excessive secretions**		A	A	V	A		
Nausea & Vomiting **Goal: Patient does not feel nauseous or vomits** • Patient verbalises if conscious		A	A	A	A		
Other symptoms (e.g. dyspnoea) a) ....N?...							
TREATMENT/PROCEDURES							
Mouth Care **Goal: Mouth is moist and clean.** • See mouth care policy • Mouth care to be given at least 4 hourly		A	A	A	A		
Micturition Difficulties **Goal: Patient is comfortable** • Urinary catheter if in retention • Urinary catheter or pads, if general weakness creates incontinence		A	A	A	A		
MEDICATION (If not appropriate record as N/A)							
Goal: All medication is given safely & accurately. • If syringe driver in progress check at least 4 hourly • If medication not required please record as N/A		A	A.	A	A		
Nurse Signature **Repeat this page 24 hrly. Spare copies on Ward**		Early SS		Late LJ		Night	

INTEGRATED CARE PATHWAY FOR THE TERMINAL/DYING PHASE

NAME: Mr Smith .... UNIT NO: 123 XYZ ...... DATE: 02.04.02

Complete **12 hourly**		08:00	20:00
MOBILITY/PRESSURE AREA CARE	**Goal: Patient is comfortable and in a safe environment** Patient is moved for comfort only with pressure relieving aids as appropriate e.g. special mattress	A	
BOWEL CARE	**Goal: Patient is not agitated or distressed due to constipation or diarhoea**	A	
PSYCHOLOGICAL/ INSIGHT SUPPORT	**Patient** **Goal: Patient becomes aware of the situation as appropriate** • Patient is informed of procedures • Touch, verbal communication is continued	A	

	Family/Other
	Goal: Family/Other are prepared for the patient's imminent
	        death with the aim of achieving peace of mind and
	        acceptance
	• Check understanding
	• Recognition of patient dying
	• Inform of measures taken to maintain patient's comfort
	• Explain possibility of physical symptoms e.g fatigue
	• Psychological symptoms such as anxiety/depression
	• Social issues such as financial implications
		V	

RELIGIOUS/SPIRITUAL SUPPORT	**Goal: Appropriate religious/spiritual support has been given**	A	
CARE OF THE FAMILY/OTHERS	**Goal: The needs of those attending the patient are** **accommodated**	A.	

IF YOU HAVE CHARTERED 'V' AGAINST ANY GOAL SO FAR, PLEASE COMPLETE VARIANCE SHEET AT THE BACK OF THE PATHWAY BEFORE SIGNING BELOW
Repeat this page each 24 hours. Spare sheets on Ward

Nurse Signature   Early .... S.S. .... Late .... Night ....
MULTIDISCIPLINARY PROGRESS NOTES

Ward round - discontinue antibiotics
                    ～～～～ SpR

2.4.02 Reviewed patient's pain, has required x 3 prn doses of
diamorphine. I would suggest commencing a syringe driver
with 15 mg of diamorphine S/C over 24°.

INTEGRATED CARE PATHWAY FOR THE TERMINAL/DYING PHASE

NAME: _Mr Smith_ .... UNIT NO: _123 XYZ_ .... DATE: _02.04.02_

VERIFICATION OF DEATH

Date of Death _02.04.02_ .... Time of Death _19.30_ ....

Persons Present _Wife + Son_ ....

Notes _Pt comfortable at time of death_ ....

....

Signature _[signature]_ .... Time Verified _20.00_ ....

CARE AFTER DEATH	**Goal 12:** GP Practice contacted re patient's death Date: _3/4/02_ Yes ☐ No ☑
	Goal 13: Procedures for laying out followed according to hospital policy Yes ☑ No ☐ • Input patients death on hospital computer
	Goal 14: Procedure following death discussed or carried out N/A ☑ Yes ☐ No ☐ (If yes please indicate) Patient had infectious disease ☐ Patient has religious needs ☐ Post mortem discussed ☐
	Goal 15: Family/other given information on hospital procedures Yes ☑ No ☐ • Hospital information booklet given to Family/Other about necessary legal tasks • Relatives/other informed to ring Bereavement Office after 10am on next working day to make an appointment to collect death certificate
	Goal 16: Hospital policy followed for patient's valuables & belongings Yes ☑ No ☐ **OUT OF OFFICE HOURS:** • Belongings listed and put in A&E Clothing Store • Valuables listed and put in A&E night safe **IN OFFICE HOURS** • Belongings & valuables listed & taken to Bereavement Office
	Goal 17: Necessary documentation & advice is given to the appropriate person Yes ☑ No ☐ • Bereavement Office Booklet Given
	Goal 18: Bereavement leaflet given Yes ☑ No ☐ • 'What to do after death' booklet given (DHSS) if applicable • Grieving leaflet given
	IF YOU HAVE CHARTED "NO" AGAINST ANY GOAL SO FAR, PLEASE COMPLETE VARIANCE SHEET AT THE BACK OF THE PATHWAY BEFORE SIGNING BELOW Nurse Signature _[signature]_ .... Date _2.4.02_ *** HAVE YOU COMPLETED THE LAST 4 & 12 HOURLY OBSERVATION**
	PLEASE CONTACT THE PALLIATIVE CARE TEAM TO INFORM THEM THAT THIS PATIENT WAS ON A PATHWAY. EXT 2274

INTEGRATED CARE PATHWAY FOR THE TERMINAL/DYING PHASE

NAME: Mr. SMITH............ UNIT NO: 123 XYZ.... DATE: 01/04/02....

VARIANCE ANALYSIS FOR TERMINAL/DYING PHASE

HOSPITAL

CONSULTANT: Dr A
DATE OF ADMISSION: 25/03/02
DATE OF DEATH: ....
WARD: X

DATE	WHAT VARIANCE OCCURRED?	WHY DID VARIANCE OCCUR?	ACTION TAKEN	INITIALS	TITLE
1.4.02	Antibiotics continued	Antibiotics for chest infection	for review by medical team	LJ	Nurse
1.4.02	unable to contact GP	surgery closed	contact GP tomorrow	LJ	Nurse
1.4.02	Patient appeared to be in pain	unable to take oral analgesia	5mg diamorphine given	LJ	Nurse
1.4.02	Patient became agitated	Agitated on change of position	Patient repositioned	LJ	Nurse
2.4.02	Patient in pain	given diamorphine 5mg stat / Pain due to primary disease	given diamorphine 5mg stat	JJ	nurse
02.04.02	Patient in pain	Cancer pain	5mg diamorphine stat given + 50 commenced - 15mg diamorphine	SS	nurse
02.04.02	Respiratory tract secretions developed	Pt unable to cough	400 mcg Hyoscine Hydrobromide given.	LJ	Nurse
02.04.02	wife distressed	Patient's imminent death	support given	SS	nurse
02.04.02	Unable to inform GP of patient's death	surgery closed	contact tomorrow	LJ	Nurse

Chapter 3

Symptom control in care of the dying

Paul Glare, Andrew Dickman, and Margaret Goodman

Section 1—Paul Glare

How can the Liverpool Integrated Care Pathway for the Dying Patient (LCP) influence symptom control?

Inadequacies have been identified in the hospital/acute care setting in the areas of symptom control and psychological support of dying patients (1). It is inappropriate to expect palliative care teams to be involved in *every* dying patient's care—in the case of Royal Liverpool University Hospitals (RLUH), the figure is approximately 15% of deaths. An integrated care pathway (ICP) provides one solution to this problem by giving the primary health care team a way to improve patients' access to high quality symptom assessment and treatment in terminal care in general. An ICP can influence symptom control by providing the multidisciplinary team with an agreed plan of care by contributing professionals that specifies goals, guideline-based interventions, and a flow sheet that outlines the expected and realistic course of the patient's care (2, 3). Furthermore, each episode can be described, tracked, and monitored to ensure that intermediate and final outcomes like symptom control are within an accepted range of quality. The ICP is a multidisciplinary document that replaces all previous documentation.

If the ICP is not followed at any point, or a specified goal is not achieved the health care professional records a reason for the deviation as a 'variance'. Analysis of this variance provides a mechanism for analysing the reasons for not achieving the desired outcomes of care and helps identify training and resource needs.

The key components of the LCP are:

(a) Identification that the patient is imminently dying, and to be included in the pathway.

(b) Initial assessment and care.

(c) Ongoing assessment.

(d) Care of the relatives after death.

At the RLUH, a patient is eligible to be commenced on the LCP if the primary health care team agrees that the patient is imminently dying and fulfils at least two of the following four conditions:

◆ Bed-bound.

◆ Semi-comatose.

◆ Only able to take sips of fluid.

◆ No longer able to take tablets.

Identifying that a patient is in the last few days of life is relatively straightforward in cancer (4) but may be harder to predict in patients with other eventually fatal illnesses, e.g. congestive heart failure, chronic obstructive pulmonary disease, or Alzheimer's disease (5).

The initial assessment has three main symptom-related goals. These are aimed at ensuring the patient's comfort and include:

(a) **Goal 1** Assessment of current medication and non-essentials discontinued.

(b) **Goal 2** The prescribing of PRN subcutaneous medication for symptom control.

(c) **Goal 3** Discontinuation of inappropriate interventions.

Drugs can be non-essential because they are given for long-term disease prevention and health maintenance (e.g. agents that alter bone and calcium metabolism; hypolipidaemic agents) and are clearly irrelevant in the last days of life. Many other drugs can be stopped because the effects of the disease they are treating or preventing is also less relevant in the last days of life, even if it occurs (e.g. antibiotics, anti-hypertensives, anti-ulcer treatment). In their place, analgesics, anti-emetics, anticholinergics, anti-convulsants, and sedatives form the new 'essential' drug list.

For drugs that need to be continued in the last few days of life, the oral route should be used if possible since some patients are able to swallow tablets right up until death. If the patient is unable to swallow, oral drugs need to be converted to the subcutaneous route and a syringe driver should be commenced if appropriate. Setting the syringe driver up within four hours of the doctor's order is a sub-goal of the LCP.

Appropriate as required (PRN) medications should be prescribed in case the patient develops further symptoms. The most common symptoms are: pain, nausea and vomiting, agitation, and respiratory tract secretions.

Aside from rationalizing medications, the other core goal of the LCP is to stop inappropriate interventions. Interventions can be medical or nursing ones and stopping them includes ensuring that a 'not for CPR' order is written in the patient's notes. Medical interventions including blood tests, antibiotics, and intravenous medications should be discontinued. Nursing interventions including taking vital signs and routine turning regimes should be discontinued or modified.

Ongoing assessment of pain and comfort measures is documented every four hours on the LCP forms. As well as symptom control, the other foci of assessment include mouth care, bowel care, pressure care, and psychological support of the patient and/or family.

What are the commonest symptoms in the dying patient?

The main symptoms in the terminal/dying phase are: pain, nausea and vomiting, agitation/restlessness, breathlessness. Other problems occurring in the last hours/days of life include: inability to swallow, constipation, urinary problems/catheterization,

Table 3.1 Common symptoms in the last 48 hours of life (adapted from references 6 and 7)

Symptom	Incidence	Poor control
Death rattle[a]	56%	0%
Pain	51–56%	1–4%
Restlessness[b]	30–42%	1.5–4%
Dyspnoea	22–26%	0–2%
Nausea and vomiting	12–14%	1–2%
Confusion	9–12%	0–6%

[a] Not reported by Turner *et al*. (7).
[b] Terminal agitation/restlessness and emotional distress reported
separately by Turner *et al*. (7), but they are combined here.

retained respiratory tract secretions, bleeding, and seizures. Surveys have indicated that by far the four most common problems are pain, nausea and vomiting, agitation, and respiratory tract secretions (6, 7) (see Table 3.1). Fortunately, these symptoms only need a handful of medications to be controlled, all of which can be given subcutaneously.

How do you manage pain in the dying patient?

Pain control is achievable in the vast majority of patients in the last few days of life using existing methods. Even in the dying phase, it is important that the four basic principles of pain (and other symptom) control are kept in mind (8):

◆ Identify and reverse (if possible) the noxious stimulus.

◆ Identify and reverse (if possible) any 'pain threshold' issues.

◆ If indicated, use opioids correctly.

◆ If appropriate, use co-analgesic medications.

1. **The first step** is to try to take a history and do a focused physical examination with the aim of trying to identify the noxious stimulus that is causing the pain. Investigations such as X-rays or neuroimaging that are commonly ordered to confirm the clinical diagnosis of the pain mechanism would not be appropriate in the dying phase, and would constitute a variance if performed. It is important to remember that pain in patients with cancer can be due to the disease, a side-effect of its treatment, debility, or unrelated causes. Debility will be commoner at this time than earlier in the illness. Myofascial pain, constipation, muscle spasm, and capsulitis of the shoulder were all debility-related pains in the 'Top10' pains experienced by patients with cancer admitted to Sobell House (9).

2. **The second step** is to do a psychosocial assessment, to try to identify any 'pain threshold' issues that are complicating the pain. This may be quite difficult to assess in the imminently dying patient and will often present as terminal agitation/restlessness (see next section).

3. **The third step** is to consider using opioids—and if they are indicated, to use them correctly, according to the standard principles (10). For patients being put on the LCP,

there are four scenarios to consider, depending on whether or not the patient has pain or not, and is already on morphine or not.

Four scenarios

1. Patient in pain and already on oral morphine or other opioid (i.e. current analgesia ineffective or there is rapid escalating pain): This constitutes a complex pain problem. The patient should be referred to the Palliative Care Service for assessment and advice about management. If the current analgesia is ineffective, options include switching opioids or adding a different adjuvant agent. If pain is escalating, increase previous opioid dose by 33–50%. Patients in the dying phase who fit this scenario would usually be converted to the subcutaneous route (see below).

2. Patient in pain, but not yet on oral morphine or other strong opioid (i.e. onset of pain in last few days of life, having not previously required analgesia): If the pain is continuous and moderate-to-severe in intensity, a strong opioid like morphine (oral route) or diamorphine (subcutaneous route) is used. At RLUH, the LCP intervention requires subcutaneous diamorphine 2.5–5 mg 4 hrly PRN. This needs to be reviewed after 24 hours and if more than two doses have been given PRN then consider starting a syringe driver over 24 hours.

3. Patient not in pain, on oral morphine or other opioid (i.e. pain controlled on stable dose of opioid): Initially the current treatment is continued and if necessary conversion to the subcutaneous route with consideration of a constant infusion via a syringe driver. If the patient needs to convert to a 24 hr subcutaneous infusion of diamorphine, divide the total daily dose of morphine by three (e.g. 30 mg sustained release oral morphine twice daily = diamorphine 20 mg via subcutaneous syringe driver). The patient also needs to have a PRN dose of diamorphine prescribed as "rescue" medication. This should be 1/6th of 24 hr dose in syringe driver (e.g. if diamorphine 20 mg subcutaneously via driver, will require 2.5–5 mg diamorphine subcutaneously 4 hrly PRN).

   If the patient needs conversion from other strong opioids to diamorphine, contact the palliative care team.

4. Patient not in pain, and not on strong opioid. Prescribe subcutaneous diamorphine 2.5–5 mg q4h PRN, for use if pain develops. This needs to be reviewed after 24 hours and if two or more doses have been required PRN then consider a syringe driver over 24 hours as above.

As with patients in the earlier stage of their illness, regular review of the level of pain relief is needed and this is directed by four hourly assessments by the ICP. It is usually not recommended to start modified release morphine preparations in the last few days of life, however, because they are variable in their absorption and are not suitable for rapid dose titration in patients with uncontrolled pain. It is reasonable to continue them while the oral route is available if the pain is controlled.

In countries where diamorphine is not available, hydromorphone or morphine tartrate have similar solubility to diamorphine. The rectal route can be used (e.g. oxycodone 30 mg suppositories every eight hours) but is less acceptable to some patients/families and is much more limited in what drugs and doses can be administered (11).

Fentanyl patches make the transdermal route an obvious alternative to oral in terminally ill patients who are unable to swallow, but there is uncertainty about their use in the dying phase. Like sustained release morphine, they should not be commenced during this period if pain develops, because of their slow onset of action and difficulty of titration. But what should one do if the patient already on a fentanyl patch develops unstable pain? It is preferable to continue the patch and use PRN diamorphine for breakthrough in the first 24 hours, changing this to a continuous infusion via a syringe driver once the requirement is established, rather than stopping the patches and trying to convert it to a different opioid. A retrospective chart review from Marie Curie Centre Liverpool, UK has compared patients continuing with transdermal fentanyl and using supplementary dose of diamorphine, with those only having diamorphine via a syringe driver (12). The total daily opioid dose in the fentanyl group was higher, but they received fewer breakthrough doses and had better pain relief. Thus it seems that continuing the patch doesn't compromise pain control in the last few days and may be associated with fewer episodes of pain and fewer breakthrough dose. It is preferred not to discontinue the fentanyl patches thereby avoiding unpredictable pain.

4. The fourth step in basic pain management is to use co-analgesic drugs for components of the pain that are not very opioid-responsive, giving due caution to polypharmacy, drug interactions, and side-effects. Administering these drugs can become problematic in patients who are unable to swallow, and the options will vary according to the local availability of different formulations. For example, for patients with bone pain, NSAID may be available as suppositories, or dexamethasone can be given subcutaneously. For muscle spasm pain, diazepam can be given rectally. Anticonvulsants and antidepressants for neuropathic pain are more of a problem: they can often be omitted for a few days even if they are required because they have long half-lives, especially in the context of hepatic or renal impairment. Subcutaneous clonazepam or ketamine may be considered as substitutes for the usual oral agents if necessary. It must always be remembered that some pains occurring in the dying phase require non-pharmacological management. Common examples include mouth care for xerostomia, a change of mattress and pressure area care for decubitus ulcers, and enemas for constipation.

How do you manage agitation in the dying patient?

Restlessness and agitation during the dying phase is a sad and distressing problem. The dissolution of autonomy and dignity associated with an agitated delirium, the associated stigma of mental illness, and the evaporation of quality of remaining life demand quick, active, and aggressive multidisciplinary palliative interventions (13). As with pain and other symptoms, the cause of agitation needs to be identified, and reversed if possible, although the precise aetiology can be identified in less than 50% cases. Again, reliance is on history taking and clinical examination rather than investigations. A single venepuncture to check electrolytes, calcium, glucose, and white cell count could be warranted. This would then be recorded as a variance on the LCP.

Commonest causes of agitation in the last days of life include drug toxicity, metabolic upset, physical causes, and anxiety/emotional distress. The syndrome of opioid toxicity that includes mental clouding has also been described (14). If a reversible cause is identified, it should be removed if possible. If opioid toxicity is suspected, opioid switching (± rehydration) can be tried, although the outcome may be difficult to evaluate in such a short time frame and IV fluids would constitute a variance to the LCP. Drug withdrawal from alcohol or benzodiazepines needs to be considered and treated. Metabolic derangement can be corrected although hyper- or hypoglycemia are probably the only ones that are worth treating in the last 48–72 hours of life. Hypoxia can respond to supplementary oxygen. Antibiotics may be warranted if there is infection and steroids if there are brain metastases. Physical discomforts are an important source of agitation/confusion that are easily remedied. A distended bladder due to urinary retention is very distressing and insertion of a urinary catheter is very effective. Similarly, evacuating a distended bowel relieves distress quickly. In a patient with anxiety and/or emotional distress, talking should always be tried before medications.

There are two main pharmacological approaches in the palliation of agitation: the use of benzodiazepines to provide sedation and the use of anti-psychotic drugs like haloperidol to provide tranquillization. In the dying phase, benzodiazepines are usually employed, because they are the mainstay of treatment for anxiety or emotional distress, and the initial management of confusion (major tranquillizers like haloperidol or levomepromazine having less of a place than prior to the onset of the dying phase). There are a variety of short- and long-acting benzodiazepines to use, but in the dying phase, midazolam is usually given, via a syringe driver (5–20 mg/24 hrs initially, titrating up to 80 mg/day or more). It can also be given by intermittent injection. Following the LCP, the medication to be prescribed depends on whether or not the patient is already restless/agitated:

(a) If the patient is currently confused, agitated, or distressed, a PRN dose of midazolam (2.5–10 mg) subcutaneously four hourly is prescribed. Review the medication usage after 24 hours; if two or more PRN dose have been given then consider a syringe driver over 24 hours, while continuing to give PRN dosage accordingly.

(b) If terminal restlessness/agitation are absent, prescribe midazolam 2.5–10 mg subcutaneously four hourly PRN. Again, review the medication usage after 24 hours; if two or more PRN dose have been given then consider a syringe driver over 24 hours, while continuing to give PRN dosage accordingly.

If symptoms persist, the palliative care team should be contacted. For the management of confusion due to drug toxicity, metabolic derangement, or altered sensorium, a major tranquillizer, e.g. haloperidol or levomepromazine, would usually be indicated. Benzodiazepines like midazolam occasionally cause paradoxical behaviour reactions. Haloperidol is usually preferred to phenothiazines by psychiatrists because of its superior side-effect profile (13), but levomepromazine or chlorpromazine have both found to be safe and effective in the dying phase in palliative care (15, 16). Haloperidol is given by oral (1.5–3 mg) or subcutaneous (1–2 mg) boluses every 30 minutes to one hour, until the patient settles. The total amount given can then be administered over 24 hours either in divided doses or in a syringe driver. Chlorpromazine or levomepromazine are more sedating than haloperidol, they cause hypotension and being phenothiazines can lower the seizure threshold. Other alternatives include the new generation atypical neuroleptics (e.g. risperidone, olanzepine) and phenobarbitone or even propofol in extreme cases (13).

In the non-pharmacological management of delirium, a safe environment needs to be provided and psychological interventions are helpful. Continuity of carers and the presence of a near relative are the most important psychological therapeutic strategies (13).

Section 2—Andrew Dickman

How do you manage respiratory tract secretions in the dying patient?

Patients approaching the terminal stages of life are often unable to clear upper respiratory tract secretions, which lead to the condition known as the 'death rattle'. In clinical practice, this is a common symptom, occurring in up to 92% of dying patients (17). Clinical experience would suggest that most patients are unconscious when terminal secretions are present and it is therefore not possible to evaluate the benefit to the patient of alleviation of the symptom of respiratory tract secretions. However, it has been suggested that terminal secretions may contribute to the development of dyspnoea and terminal restlessness. No association has been demonstrated between level of hydration and terminal secretions (18). The most apparent benefit of control of respiratory tract secretions is to minimize the distress of relatives and carers.

Treatment of this condition can involve positional changes and pharmacological intervention; difficult cases may require suction. Not all patients will be suitable for positional changes, which involves moving to a position so as to facilitate secretion drainage. Suction may be unpleasant and the patient may require a subcutaneous dose of midazolam (e.g. 2.5–5 mg) prior to the procedure. The main treatment of terminal secretions, therefore, involves the antimuscarinic drugs.

One important point to remember about antimuscarinic drugs is that in general they will not control or diminish secretions that are well established. Treatment must be started as soon as symptoms become apparent. There are currently three antimuscarinic drugs used to treat respiratory tract secretions in the UK: hyoscine hydrobromide, glycopyrronium, and hyoscine butylbromide (see Table 3.2). It is surprising that given the relatively common nature of this symptom, there is a paucity of evidence to support the superiority of any of these drugs. One small study concluded that there was no clear difference between the three (19). However, glycopyrronium is almost one-and-a-half times as potent as hyoscine hydrobromide in preventing salivary secretions, a component of terminal secretions (20). Glycopyrronium is less expensive than hyoscine hydrobromide and has become the drug of choice in many centres. Hyoscine butylbromide is the least expensive of the three, but its use in the treatment of terminal secretions is not widespread.

Both glycopyrronium and hyoscine butylbromide are quaternary ammonium compounds. This means that neither penetrates the blood brain barrier easily due to the bulky size. Consequently, these drugs are devoid of the sedative and direct anti-emetic

Table 3.2 Antimuscarinic drug comparisons

	Hyoscine hydrobromide	Glycopyrronium	Hyoscine-n-butylbromide
Ampoule size	400 μg/ml	600 μg/ml	20 mg/ml
Cost (per ampoule)[a]	£2.81	92 p	19 p
Usual daily dose range	1.2–2.4 mg	0.6–1.2 mg	20–60 mg[b]
Daily cost	£8.43–16.86	£0.92–1.82	£0.19–0.57

[a] National Health Service (UK) prices (August 2001).
[b] May need to use doses up to 120 mg to control secretions (costing £1.14 daily).

effects associated with hyoscine hydrobromide. All three drugs may be administered subcutaneously by injection or via a continuous subcutaneous infusion. Hyoscine hydrobromide can be administered via a transdermal patch and has been nebulized to treat terminal secretions (21) but its use in this manner cannot generally be recommended. Doses and costs of these drugs are shown in Table 3.2.

How do you manage dyspnoea in the dying patient?

Like pain, dyspnoea is a subjective experience involving several factors that influence the degree and perception. As the patient enters the terminal phase it may not be possible or practical to address all of these causes. The aim of treatment changes to focus on the perception of breathlessness and any associated anxiety, ensuring the patient remains comfortable.

Pharmacological intervention forms the mainstay of treatment, although non-drug measures, such as a cool air or a calming hand, may still have a role. Typical pharmacological regimens involve opioids, benzodiazepines, and oxygen. Consideration may also be given to anticholinergic drugs and phenothiazines. As the patient becomes progressively weaker, oral administration of medication may no longer be possible and drugs are commonly given via the subcutaneous route. The rectal route can be used, although suitable preparations do not exist for all drugs.

Oxygen may be used for hypoxic patients, although the evidence is weak (22). If the patient is unconscious, consideration to discontinue this treatment can be made. Patients with dyspnoea typically experience tachypnoea and anxiety. It is believed that by reducing the respiratory rate and addressing the associated anxiety, the perception of breathlessness is also reduced. The opioids act in a variety of ways; essentially they can reduce the respiratory rate and reduce the level of anxiety. Morphine or diamorphine can be administered via subcutaneous injection or infusion. The dose used depends upon previous oral requirements, although for an opioid naïve patient a suitable starting dose would be 10 mg of morphine daily. If the patient has been receiving opioids for pain, the dose can be increased to achieve the necessary reduction in respiratory rate to a level of 15 breaths per minute. This may require a dose increase of up to 50% (22). Nebulized morphine has been used in the palliative treatment of dyspnoea with varying results. Until more positive evidence is forthcoming, this route of administration cannot be recommended (23).

Benzodiazepines are also a useful treatment and are indicated for dyspnoea associated with anxiety. Midazolam via subcutaneous injection or infusion is the drug of choice. Stat doses of 5–10 mg may be given and a continuous infusion of 10–30 mg is suggested. Occasionally, lorazepam is given sublingually at a dose of 0.5–1 mg up to four times daily.

The phenothiazine, levomepromazine, is anxiolytic and can be used to treat dyspnoea associated with anxiety or agitation. A suitable starting dose would be 12.5 mg daily via subcutaneous injection or infusion. Other phenothiazines should not be administered this way, although promethazine is occasionally used (24).

Terminal secretions may contribute to the development of terminal dyspnoea, although evidence is lacking. Nonetheless, an anticholinergic drug, such as glycopyrronium, should be started as soon as terminal secretions become apparent.

No patient should believe that they will die suffering from dyspnoea. Although opioids and sedatives are employed, the aim of treatment is to reduce the level of anxiety and improve the sensation of breathlessness, whilst maintaining the patient's level of consciousness. However, this may not always be possible; indeed as the patient becomes weaker, drowsiness becomes more apparent. This should be explained clearly to the patient and their relatives or carers.

What are the benefits of using a syringe driver to deliver subcutaneous medication?

The syringe driver is a portable battery-operated device that can be used to deliver a continuous subcutaneous infusion. There are currently two types of SIMS Graseby® syringe driver suitable for use: the MS26 and MS16A (see Figure 3.1).

The MS26 is probably the simplest to use and is therefore recommended in the palliative care setting. The administration of drugs via a continuous subcutaneous infusion (CSCI) has been shown to be common practice within specialist palliative care units across the UK and Eire (25).

However, the use of CSCIs is not solely limited to palliative care; they have been used successfully in a variety of conditions, such as thalassaemia, myasthenia gravis, and Parkinson's disease.

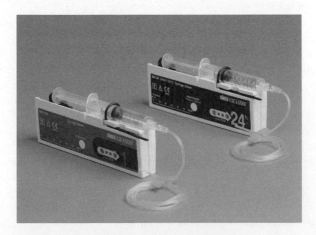

Figure 3.1 The SIMS Graseby MS16A (left) and MS26 (right).

The condition of an advanced cancer patient is likely to deteriorate, such that parenteral administration of drugs may become necessary. Regular intramuscular or subcutaneous injections are painful; the rectal route is not always appropriate or acceptable; intravenous injections require access and needlessly increase the risk of infection. The use of a syringe driver to deliver a CSCI of drugs allows improved symptom control with less discomfort and inconvenience. Indeed, a CSCI is as effective as an intravenous infusion. A CSCI is often suggested to treat symptoms in the last few days of life, although it is not restricted to this indication. A single CSCI containing up to three drugs will control the vast majority of symptoms that a dying patient is likely to experience. In exceptional circumstances four or five drugs may be required, and specialist palliative care advice in such circumstances is recommended to review medication and advise on drug compatibilities.

The main uses for the syringe driver are shown in Table 3.3.

Table 3.3 Indications for subcutaneous route of administration using a syringe driver in preference to other routes

Oral	Rectal	IV/IM
Nausea and vomiting	Diarrhoea	Cachexia
Dysphagia	Bowel obstruction	Fear
Severe weakness Patient preference Unconsciousness	Patient preference	Discomfort

A CSCI is extremely beneficial in the hospital, hospice, and home setting. The advantages are shown in Table 3.4.

Table 3.4 Advantages of the syringe driver

1. Increased patient comfort.

2. Control of multiple symptoms with a combination of drugs.

3. Plasma drug concentrations are maintained without peaks and troughs.

4. Independence and mobility maintained because the device is lightweight and can be worn in a holster either under or over clothes.

5. Generally needs to be assembled every 24 hours.

In addition it is important to realize that the syringe driver does not represent the fourth step of the analgesic ladder. This is a common misconception in the UK. It is vital that the patient and their family or carers are involved in the decision to start a syringe driver. There is a perception among the general public that if a patient has a syringe driver then they must be near to death, or even that the syringe driver may hasten death.

What are the practicalities of using a syringe driver?

The MS26 can deliver a max length of 60 mm over 24 hours. Since the rate of delivery is determined by **length**, greater flexibility can be achieved in the choice and brand of syringe selected. The largest Luer lok™ syringe that will attach to the driver has a volume of approximately 30 ml; a barrel length of 60 mm equates to approximately 20 ml with this size syringe. The MS26 delivers at a rate set in *mm per 24 hours*. The set up procedure is shown in Table 3.5.

Table 3.5 Procedure for setting up the MS26 syringe driver

1. Fill the syringe with drugs and dilute mixture to a maximum length of 60 mm. Use the millimetre scale on the driver for reference.
2. Prime the infusion line if required.
3. Measure length of barrel against the millimetre scale on the syringe driver.
4. Set the delivery rate. For infusion times of 24 hours, the length of the barrel represents the infusion rate. For a 12 hourly infusion, the infusion time is obtained by multiplying the length by two.
5. Attach the syringe to the driver by aligning the flange of the syringe into the slot provided on the syringe driver and secure the syringe firmly with the rubber strap.
6. Insert the battery. An audible alarm sounds. This is the noise the device makes when: • The infusion has ended. • The line is blocked. • The start/boost button is depressed for 10 seconds.

Press the start button to silence the alarm and to activate the driver. If the light on the front of the driver does not flash every 25 seconds, replace the battery.

The infusion should be sited in subcutaneous tissue, usually the chest wall in ambulant patients. Occasionally, the abdomen, upper arm, or thigh may be used. In bed-bound patients, the upper arm or thigh may occasionally be used. The scapula is a suitable infusion site in agitated patients.

What drugs can be used in a syringe driver?

As the patient approaches the terminal stages of life, it is important to review all medication. A pharmacist can provide useful advice regarding drugs that can be safely discontinued and help with the development of a new treatment strategy. Drugs previously considered essential, e.g. cardiac drugs, tamoxifen, bicalutamide, sulfonylureas, etc. should be discontinued. Several treatments can be continued via a CSCI. Indeed, a recent study found that as many as 29 different drugs were being administered via CSCI in adult specialist palliative care units throughout the UK and Eire (25). Nonetheless, most symptoms that a patient is likely to experience during the terminal phase can be adequately controlled with a combination of up to three drugs administered via a CSCI (see Table 3.6).

Analgesics

Diamorphine is the opioid of choice in the UK due to its solubility; 1 g of diamorphine dissolves in only 1.6 ml of water, compared with 21 ml for the equivalent amount of morphine sulfate. The dose to administer depends upon previous opioid requirements. Common opioid conversion factors are shown in Table 3.7.

Note that equianalgesic doses are difficult to determine and initial dose conversions should be conservative. Aim for the lowest equianalgesic dose if a range is stated; it is safer to under-dose the patient and use rescue medication for any shortfalls. A suitable dose for an opioid naïve patient would be 5–10 mg diamorphine over 24 hours.

Table 3.6 Principal drugs for administration via CSCI

Analgesic dose	Anti-emetic dose	Sedative dose	Antimuscarinic dose
Diamorphine (or morphine)	Cyclizine 100–150 mg daily	Midazolam 10–100 mg daily	Glycopyrronium 0.6–2.4 mg
Depends upon prior opioid use	Metoclopramide 30–120 mg daily	Levomepromazine 25–200 mg daily	Hyoscine butylbromide 60–180 mg
	Dimenhydrinate 50–200 mg daily	Haloperidol 10–30 mg daily	Hyoscine hydrobromide 1.2–2.4 mg
	Levomepromazine 6.25–25 mg daily		
	Haloperidol 5–10 mg daily		

Table 3.7 Equianalgesic factors of common opioids (adapted from ref. 7)

Opioid	Conversion factor to subcutaneous diamorphine (mg)[a]
Codeine (oral)	0.04
Diamorphine (oral)	0.33
Fentanyl (72 hour transdermal dose)	See text
Hydromorphone (oral)	2.5
Morphine (oral)	0.33
Morphine (parenteral)	0.66–1.0
Oxycodone (oral)	0.66

[a] To calculate the dose, multiply the dose of opioid (in milligrams) by the conversion factor. For example, 120 mg morphine $\times$ 3 = 40 mg diamorphine.

Should the patient be currently using a fentanyl patch, it is sensible to continue with this. A four hourly rescue dose of subcutaneous diamorphine should be given to treat breakthrough pain. Refer to Table 3.8 to determine suitable rescue doses.

After 24 hours, the total number of rescue doses should be totalled and administered via a CSCI, in addition to the fentanyl patch.

Table 3.8 Determination of rescue doses of diamorphine for patients using a fentanyl patch

Fentanyl patch strength	24 hour diamorphine dose	Four hourly rescue dose of diamorphine
25 µg/hour	30 mg	5 mg
50 µg/hour	60 mg	10 mg
75 µg/hour	90 mg	15 mg
100 µg/hour	120 mg	20 mg

For example, consider a patient currently prescribed a fentanyl '50' patch. This is equivalent to 60 mg of diamorphine. The four hourly rescue dose of diamorphine via subcutaneous injection would be 10 mg. If the patient required three rescue doses in a 24 hour period, 30 mg of diamorphine would then be added to a CSCI. This is *in addition* to the patch. The new four hourly rescue dose would be 15 mg diamorphine.

Diamorphine is compatible with all the drugs shown in Table 3.6, although problems can arise with cyclizine. Diamorphine hydrochloride and cyclizine lactate mixtures are chemically and physically stable in water for injections up to concentrations of 20 mg/ml over 24 hours. If the diamorphine concentration exceeds 20 mg/ml, crystallization may occur unless the concentration of cyclizine is *no greater than* 10 mg/ml. Similarly, if the concentration of cyclizine exceeds 20 mg/ml, crystallization may occur unless the concentration of diamorphine is *no greater than* 15 mg/ml (24).

Anti-emetics

Nausea and vomiting is an unpleasant symptom to experience and prompt action to control it is essential. A thorough assessment and history is vital in order to identify the cause(s) so as to enable the most suitable choice of anti-emetic. However, this is not always possible. In cases where a cause cannot be identified, the use of a broad-spectrum anti-emetic is suggested. In the UK, cyclizine is usually prescribed (a suitable choice in the USA would be dimenhydrinate) (24). If cyclizine does not work, levomepromazine should be considered.

Cyclizine and dimenhydrinate are antihistamines that exhibit additional antimuscarinic activity. These properties give these drugs their broad anti-emetic action, with the main action sited within the vomiting centre. In cases of large-volume vomiting due to bowel obstruction, cyclizine (but *not* dimenhydrinate) may be combined with the antimuscarinic, glycopyrronium. Cyclizine occasionally crystallizes with hyoscine butylbromide, so this combination should be avoided. Any mixtures containing cyclizine must be diluted with water for injections to prevent incompatibilities. Unwanted effects of cyclizine and dimenhydrinate include drowsiness and dry mouth. Rarely, cyclizine may exacerbate severe congestive heart failure and may occasionally cause irritation at the infusion site.

Metoclopramide and haloperidol are dopamine antagonists. They are particularly useful if nausea and vomiting is due to drugs or a homeostatic disorder (e.g. renal failure, hypercalcaemia). In addition, metoclopramide is prokinetic and is useful if gastric stasis is believed to be the cause of nausea and vomiting.

Antimuscarinic drugs have already been discussed above in the treatment of terminal secretions. The antimuscarinics can also be used to treat bowel colic and large-volume vomiting.

Levomepromazine is an anti-emetic that acts at the key sites in the vomiting pathway. It is therefore an effective anti-emetic for use in palliative care. However, it is not used first-line because of its principal adverse effect of sedation. This is used beneficially, though, in terminal restlessness (see below). Like cyclizine, levomepromazine can cause irritation at the infusion site. Levomepromazine can be mixed with all drugs shown in Table 3.6.

Sedatives

Midazolam is the drug of choice for terminal restlessness. It is compatible with all drugs in Table 3.6 (except dimenhydrinate). Midazolam is particularly useful for terminal restlessness that may be associated with anguish or anxiety. Resistant cases, particularly patients who are confused and agitated, possibly with paranoid thoughts, may need the addition of levomepromazine or haloperidol. High doses of these drugs should not be used without the use of midazolam in patients with brain tumours due to the increased risk of seizures.

Section 3—Margaret Goodman

Deciding to discontinue nursing interventions

When it becomes apparent that the patient's condition has reached the stage where there is no doubt that death is imminent there is a need to redefine the goals of the care to be provided. Essentially the patient will be weak, bed-bound, drowsy for long periods, may be disoriented with an increasing disinterest in food and fluid and in what is happening around him/her, and finding it difficult to swallow medications. Given this scenario it is necessary to be sure that any nursing interventions are appropriate and those that will not contribute to an easeful death are withdrawn. In essence all nursing interventions should now be focused on comfort and safety.

As it is difficult to predict when a patient will die, there is a need to balance the interventions which can safely be withdrawn without giving rise to the prospect of additional problems should the patient survive for many days rather than only a matter of hours. There are elements of care which can readily be eliminated as they are obviously making no contribution to the patient's comfort and have simply assisted the caring team to monitor his/her condition. No useful purpose will be served by continuing to take and record vital signs or even to maintain a fluid balance record. Regular discussion with the patient and/or family by the nursing team of the patient's condition will ensure that there is sufficient information to continue an ongoing assessment of the patient's care needs and the effectiveness of any interventions that are continued. Those interventions, which should not be discontinued, will include ones concerned with elimination, mouth care, and pressure area care.

Any records that are maintained should be to eliminate the possibility of an omission of necessary interventions only. The care pathway documentation should be sufficient for this purpose.

Mouth care

One of the main consequences of a loss of interest in taking oral fluids and consequent dehydration is a dry mouth. The current view is that the dehydration associated with the terminal phase is not distressing and that hydration may be detrimental (22). The mouth is vital to the maintenance of oral communication and breathing and any problems with the mouth will result in unnecessary additional distress and suffering especially if a dry mouth prevents the patient from being able to speak to his/her family and friends.

The principles of mouth care for the dying patient are essentially the same as for any other patient and are aimed at keeping the mouth moist and clean. The major difference is that the patient is unlikely to be able, or want, to take active measures to remedy the situation for his or herself. This means that it is essential for mouth care to be provided by a nurse or other carer.

It is one nursing intervention that can be readily devolved to a family carer. This may help to give them a sense of being able to do something constructive during the final phase of their loved one's life. If family carers wish to be involved in a patient's mouth care it is important that they are taught the basic functions of the care and that regular unobtrusive reassessments of the effectiveness of the care being given are made to ensure that the patient's comfort is maintained.

The type of care necessary will depend on the status of the patient but all dying patients will require assistance to preserve a moist and clean mouth. Assessment is essential and for the terminal patient should focus primarily on how much and what type of assistance the patient requires. Evidence shows that the frequency of mouth care is more important for the maintenance of comfort than either the method of care or the type of fluid used (26). Patients who are either on continuous oxygen therapy, are mouth breathing, or unconscious require hourly or more frequent interventions for the maintenance of moist and clean mouths. Two hourly mouth care will reduce the risk of problems and increase patient comfort (27). The omission of any type of oral care for between two and four hours will significantly reduce the benefits previously achieved by oral care (28).

As long as the patient is able it is preferable that s/he is assisted in the maintenance of his or her own oral hygiene. The provision of regular drinks and giving assistance with tooth brushing can do this. A soft electric toothbrush may be helpful, but there is insufficient evidence to date to support this option. Frequent sips of water, chips of ice to suck, and small chunks of pineapple (in juice not syrup) will all help in keeping a patient's mouth moist and clean. The regular application of Vaseline or a lip salve will help in the maintenance of moist lips and reduce the risk of cracking and associated discomfort and difficulty in talking.

Current evidence indicates that the use of a soft toothbrush and toothpaste are the best tools to use to carry out effective mouth care. However as many nurses find it easier to use either foam swabs or gauze (29) it is likely that more regular and effective care will be achieved by using these tools unless the nurses involved in the care are proficient in the use of toothbrushes with patients.

The use of mouthwashes may not be appropriate for the dying patient, but where it is possible and a patient is able to tolerate them the type used should be based on patient choice. The efficacy of a mouthwash is achieved from the mechanical action rather than the fluid itself. Recent evidence indicates that normal saline is probably as effective as any other type of solution (27). An alternative for patients who are unable to rinse effectively themselves is to squirt small amount of fluid into the mouth via a syringe, though care must obviously be taken to avoid causing choking.

Saliva substitutes can be used to relieve dryness but most have a short duration of effectiveness and patient preference is for water (30).

Oral care is essential for the maintenance of patient comfort and to enable the dying patient to retain an ability to talk with those closest to him or her. The most effective means of maintaining a moist and clean mouth is by very regular oral care, i.e. no less than two hourly intervals; and giving the patient the opportunity to have a mouth moisture boost in which ever form the patient prefers, e.g. sips of water, ice chips, or small pieces of pineapple.

Table 3.9 Summary points—mouth care

1.	Mouth care is vital for the maintenance of oral communication and breathing.
2.	Mouth problems will cause unnecessary additional suffering and distress and may hinder relationships between a patient and those closest to him/her.
3.	Assessment should focus on how much and what type of assistance a patient needs.
4.	Frequency of mouth care is more important for the maintenance of comfort than either the method of care or type of fluid used.
5.	Moisture boosts at a minimum of hourly intervals are essential for patients who are mouth breathing, on oxygen therapy, or unconscious.

Micturition difficulties

Urinary dysfunction, either retention or incontinence, has been observed in over 50% of patients during the last 48 hours of life (22). Retention of urine is a little less likely than incontinence, but either problem may cause additional distress for the patient and his/her carers. Urinary output is said to decrease as death approaches and is one of the reasons why terminal dehydration may be of benefit (22). The effect of a decrease in urinary output reduces the need for bedpans, limits the distress of incontinence and the need for catheterization. Although there is no justification for maintaining a fluid balance chart, it may be useful to note how often urine is being passed. This may assist the team in deciding the ongoing management of micturition problems and in decisions regarding the use of in-dwelling urinary catheters.

Urinary retention

The possibility of urinary retention should be considered when a dying patient is restless. Constipation can also be the cause of urinary retention and in this situation it is useless to relieve retention without also relieving the constipation. For any patient with lower abdominal disease the possibility of the cancer causing a direct effect on the bladder must be considered. It is likely that this type of effect will be observed before the patient reaches the terminal phase but the possibility should remain a consideration and form part of the ongoing assessment of care needs.

When a patient is in retention it remains essential to relieve the immediate problem, but it may not always be necessary to leave the catheter *in situ* just because the patient is dying.

Urinary incontinence

Urinary incontinence may arise as a result of generalized weakness and an inability of the patient to recognize or respond to the sensation of a full bladder. In addition neurological disturbances or again the pressure of tumour in or on the bladder may result in incontinence. Some patients may experience frequency of micturition as an effect of bladder irritation from infection or tumour which may appear as incontinence.

Incontinence can be managed by the use of pads if this is acceptable to the patient and the regular changing of them does not cause additional discomfort.

The question of whether or not to catheterize a dying patient is dependent on a number of factors and the type of micturition problem. Catheterization is used to

Table 3.10 Summary points—micturition difficulties

1. Micturition difficulties of any type are distressing for a dying patient though urinary output will diminish as death approaches.

2. Retention of urine is less likely than urinary incontinence, but either problem is common in the last 48 hours of life.

3. Retention should be considered when a patient is restless. It may be an effect of either constipation or lower abdominal disease.

4. Catheterization will relieve difficulties of micturition but can be as equally distressing to patients as either retention or incontinence. Patient preference is paramount.

5. Incontinence can be managed by the use of pads if this is acceptable to the patient.

relieve the problems of retention and incontinence for the dying patient. Careful judgement should be used to ensure that the insertion of a urinary catheter will not cause additional distress and discomfort, especially when it can be anticipated that urinary output will diminish even further as death approaches. Catheterization will of course relieve retention and keep the incontinent patient dry but it should be remembered that some patients do not find a catheter comfortable and may cause as much distress as the micturition problem it is designed to solve.

Bowel care

Bowel care during the dying phase should be focused on the alleviation of new symptoms rather than having to alleviate existing problems.

Bowel management during the preceding days and week should be sufficiently robust to ensure that the patient is neither constipated nor has diarrhoea. However as the patient's condition deteriorates bowel activity will diminish and the prospect of constipation, with or without overflow is more likely. Irritation of the bowel by tumour, radiotherapy, or drugs may sometimes result in diarrhoea.

It is inappropriate to consider any bowel intervention unless the patient displays signs or symptoms of a problem. Any problems that do present should be managed to relieve them with the minimum of discomfort for the patient. Constipation can cause agitation and/or urinary retention and thorough assessment of the patient is essential to obtain the correct diagnosis. Similarly any patient with diarrhoea should be assessed to ensure that it is not constipation with overflow diarrhoea. Gentle rectal and abdominal examination should be sufficient at this stage of the patient's illness.

If a patient is constipated and distressed then a rapid resolution of the problem is essential. Although rectal laxatives are not the treatment of choice in palliative care they are the only realistic option available. This is because their action is relatively fast and to a certain extent can be controlled and will not be totally dependent on other gut activity. Stimulant suppositories, such as bisacodyl are likely to be the most effective although osmotic preparations, such as the micro-enema or Flecter's phosphate enema should be effective if the rectum is loaded. Gentle abdominal massage may assist the process. It is important to remember that any type of rectal intervention is distressing and should only be used if the patient is very distressed and it is certain that constipation is the cause of this distress.

The management of diarrhoea is primarily concerned with keeping the patient as clean and comfortable as possible. The administration of additional drugs to relieve

Table 3.11 Summary points—bowel care

1. It is inappropriate to consider any bowel intervention unless a dying patient is obviously distressed by either constipation or diarrhoea.

2. Patient agitation can be a sign of constipation.

3. Assessment of patients with diarrhoea should eliminate the possibility of constipation with overflow diarrhoea.

4. Assessment by very gentle rectal examination and abdominal palpation will be sufficient to confirm the diagnosis.

5. Rectal laxatives are the only realistic option for the essential rapid resolution of constipation in a dying patient.

6. Keeping the patient comfortable and clean is the focus for the management of diarrhoea.

diarrhoea will not usually be possible at this stage but could be attempted if the patient is able to tolerate them. Again the gradual slowing of gut activity as the patient's condition deteriorates will cause a lessening, and for many patients cessation, of the diarrhoea. Keeping the patient clean and comfortable in the presence of diarrhoea can be difficult if movement disturbs him/her. Pads should be positioned in such a way as to minimize the amount of disturbance when they are changed. This may require layering of pads so that individual pads can be removed simply by levering the patient rather than having to move or turn the patient. Charcoal pads placed strategically in the bed will assist in reducing odour and contribute to the overall comfort.

Mobility/pressure area care

Strategies for the prevention of pressure sores should have been clearly identified and implemented for individual patients prior to them entering the terminal phase. For the dying patient the promotion of dignity and comfort is paramount whilst at the same time there is a need to balance appropriate care with the patient's wishes.

All dying patients are at particular risk of skin breakdown as their deteriorating condition is accompanied by reducing mobility and cachexia. The degree of risk will to some extent depend on the speed of deterioration but will also be affected by the nature of disease and the level of existing debility. It is unrealistic to expect healing of pressure sores but the use of appropriate pressure relieving aids should help to diminish the possibility of the development of further sores or exacerbation of existing ones.

It is therefore essential that careful monitoring of the level of risk for an individual patient continues in a regular and systematic way and at each change in condition. This means that there will be a full reassessment of pressure area care at the time it is agreed that a patient should go onto the (LCP). Part of this assessment will recognize that comfort may best be promoted by confining any movement or turning of the patient other than those which are absolutely essential, for example to change soiled linen or to change position to ease breathing. Care does need to be taken to ensure that pain and discomfort from existing sores or developing ones is not exacerbated by the stopping of turns or failure to use pressure relieving aids. The tilting of a patient at slight (30°) angle has been found to be particularly effective in reducing the occurrence of sores over the hips (31).

Table 3.12 Summary points—pressure area care/mobility

1. All dying patients will be at high risk of skin breakdown.
2. Assessment should include consideration that the dignity and comfort of a patient may be best promoted by confining any turning or moving to that which is absolutely essential.
3. Care should focus on the prevention of further exacerbation of existing sores and the development of new ones. This may include the use of different pressure relieving measures/aids.
4. Suboptimal pressure care management may have to be accepted if a patient's wishes and comfort are to be accommodated.

There is no pressure sore assessment tool specific to either palliative care or the dying patient. The nurse should continue to use whichever assessment they would normally use for a bed-bound patient. Whichever tool is used, it is unlikely that a dying patient will not fall into the high or very high-risk category and will therefore 'qualify' for the use of pressure relieving aids to promote comfort.

Patients who are not already being nursed on a pressure relieving mattress will benefit from being transferred onto one at the earliest opportunity once a decision has been made to limit or stop turning. Assessment of the type of bed coverings to be used will be necessary so that skin can be kept as clean and dry as possible and reduce the potential for sweating by the avoidance of plastic draw sheets and incontinence pads.

It may be difficult for some nurses to accept that there may be some further loss of skin integrity by the adoption of these measures. The most important element of care at this time is to maintain comfort and if turning the patient to relieve pressure causes distress then it should be avoided unless by moving the patient additional comfort can be achieved.

References

1. **The SUPPORT Principal Investigators.** (1995). A controlled trial to improve care for seriously ill hospitalized patients. The Study to Understand Prognoses and Preferences for Outcomes and Risks of Treatment (SUPPORT). *J. Am. Med. Assoc.*, **274**, 1591–8.

2. **Ellershaw, J., Foster, A., Murphy, D., Shea, T., and Overill, S.** (1997). Developing an integrated care pathway for the dying patient. *Eur. J. Palliat. Care*, **4**, 203–7.

3. **Overill, S.** (1998). A practical guide to clinical pathways. *J. Integrated Care*, **2**, 93–8.

4. **Ellershaw, J. E., Sutcliffe, J. M., and Saunders, C. M.** (1995). Dehydration and the dying patient. *J. Pain Symptom Manage.*, **10**, 192–7.

5. **Finucane, T. E.** (1999). How gravely ill becomes dying. A key to end-of-life care (edit). *J. Am. Med. Assoc.*, **282**, 1670–2.

6. **Lichter, I. and Hunt, E.** (1990). The last 48 hours of life. *J. Palliat. Care*, **6**(4), 7–15.

7. **Turner, K., Chye, R., Aggarwal, G., Philip, J., Skeels, A., and Lickiss, J. N.** (1996). Dignity in dying: a preliminary study of patients in the last three days of life. *J. Palliat. Care*, **12**(2), 7–13.

8. **Virik, K. and Glare, P.** (2000). Pain management in palliative care. Reviewing the issues. *Aust. Fam. Physician*, **29**, 1027–33.

9. **Twycross, R. G. and Lack, S. A.** (1990). *Therapeutics in terminal cancer* (2nd edn). Churchill Livingstone, Edinburgh.

10. Hanks, G. W., de Conno, F., Cherny, N., *et al.* (2001). Morphine and alternative opioids in cancer pain. The EAPC recommendations. *Br. J. Cancer*, **84**, 587–93.

11. Adam, J. (1998). The last 48 hours. In *ABC of palliative care* (ed. M. Fallon and B. O'Neill), pp. 39–42. BMJ Books, London.

12. Ellershaw, J. E., Kinder, C., Aldridge, J., Allison, M., Smith, J. C. (2002) Care of the dying: is pain control compromised or enhanced by continuation of the fentanyl transdermal patch in the dying phase? *J. Pain Symptom Manage.*, **24**(4), 398–403.

13. Macleod, A. D. (1997). The management of delirium in hospice practice. *Eur. J. Palliat. Med.*, **4**, 116–20.

14. Bruera, E., Franco, J. J., Maltoni, M., *et al.* (1995). Changing patterns of agitated impaired mental status in patients with advanced cancer: associated with cognitive monitoring, rehydration and opiate rotation. *J. Pain Symptom Manage.*, **10**, 287–91.

15. West, T. (1995). Care of the dying patient. In *Oxford textbook of oncology* (ed. M. Peckham, H. Pinedo, and U. Veronesi), pp. 2439–47. Oxford University Press, Oxford.

16. McIver, B., Walsh, D., and Nelson, K. (1994). The use of chlorpromazine for symptom control in dying cancer patients. *J. Pain Symptom Manage.*, **9**, 341–5.

17. Bennett, M. I. (1996). Death rattle: An audit of hyoscine (scopolamine) use and review of management. *J. Pain Symptom Manage.*, **12**, 229–33.

18. Ellershaw, J. E., Sutcliffe, J. M., and Saunders, C. M. (1995). Dehydration and the dying patient. *J. Pain Symptom Manage.*, **10**, 192–7.

19. Hughes, A., Wilcock, A., Corcoran, R., Lucas, V., and King, A. (2000). Audit of three antimuscarinic drugs for managing retained secretions. *Palliat. Med.*, **14**, 221–2.

20. Back, I. N., Jenkins, K., Blower, A., and Beckhelling, J. (2001). A study comparing hyoscine hydrobromide and glycopyrronium in the treatment of death rattle. *Palliat. Med.*, **15**, 329–36.

21. Doyle, J., Walker, P., and Bruera, E. (2000). Nebulized scopolamine. *J. Pain Symptom Manage.*, **19**, 327–8.

22. Twycross, R. and Lichter, I. (1993). In *Oxford textbook of palliative medicine* (ed. D. Doyle, G. Hanks, and N. MacDonald), Chapter 13. Oxford Medical Publications, Oxford.

23. Zeppetella, G. (1998). The palliation of dyspnoea in terminal disease. *Am. J. Hosp. Palliat. Care*, **15**(6), 322–30.

24. Dickman, A., Varga, J., and Littlewood, C. (2000). *The syringe driver: Continuous subcutaneous infusions in palliative care* (1st edn). Oxford University Press, Oxford.

25. O'Doherty, C. A., Hall, E. J., Schofield, L., and Zeppetella, G. (2001). Drugs and syringe drivers: a survey of adult specialist palliative care practice in the United Kingdom and Eire. *Palliat. Med.*, **15**, 149–54.

26. Duxbury, A., Thakker, N., and Wastell, D. (1989). A double-blind crossover trial of a mucin-containing artificial saliva. *Br. Dent. J.*, **166**, 115–20.

27. Homes, S. (1996). Nursing management of oral care in older patients. *Nurs. Times*, **92**, 37–8.

28. Howarth, H. (1997). Mouth care procedures for the very ill. *Nurs. Times*, **93**, 345–55.

29. Krishnasamy, M. (1995). Oral problems in advanced cancer. *Eur. J. Cancer Care*, **4**, 173–7.

30. Miller, M. and Kearney, N. (2001). Oral care for patients with cancer: A review of the literature. *Cancer Nurs.*, **24**, 241–4.

31. Seilor, W., Allen, S., and Stahelin, H. (1986). Influence of the 30 degree laterally inclined position and the 'super-soft' 3 piece mattress on skin oxygen tension on areas of maximum pressure—implications for pressure sore prevention. *Gerontology*, **32**, 158–66.

Chapter 4

Ethical issues in care of the dying

Andrew Thorns and Eve Garrard

How can the Liverpool Care Pathway for the Dying Patient (LCP) influence ethical decision making?

The aim of care pathways is to promote the principle of high quality care and this applies to ethical issues just as much as to other aspects of patient and family care.

Health care professionals frequently find themselves trying to make difficult ethical decisions at the end of life. The right course of action may not be clear, leaving professionals anxious that morally or legally they are acting inappropriately, for example in connection with potentially difficult decisions about withholding or withdrawing treatments, or about the use of sedation or analgesia for symptom control. The failure to address such issues adequately can interfere with good patient care if it leads to the patient continuing burdensome treatments or being denied the relief of discomfort. So it is important to monitor ethical decisions, show how they are justified, and continuously aim to improve them.

The patient, relatives, and friends may also be concerned about these ethical issues as a result of coverage by the media. They will want both reassurance that the health care team is acting correctly and the opportunity for discussion. In order to meet these needs health care professionals have to be confident of their own position. The LCP makes it possible to incorporate available evidence and national or regional policies to promote good practice. When difficult decisions are required the health care professional can then feel reassured both in moral as well as in legal terms.

Advice contained in the LCP can only be presented in general terms and it is vital to recognize that the decision making process has to be tailored to the individual situation. The information contained in this chapter, when used alongside the LCP, can facilitate this process, but must be supplemented by sensitivity to the details of the particular situation in which decisions have to be taken. Good communication skills in these situations is of the first importance. The correct moral action may at times be clear, but communicating such decisions in highly emotive situations is often difficult. As the complexity of a situation increases, so the need for skilled communication increases too, and this often requires the careful exploration of ideas, concerns, and expectations, followed by lengthy discussion and negotiation. There is little point in arriving at the correct moral decision if the necessary skills are not available to communicate this to those involved.

Ethical framework

What is the best approach to ethical decision making?

A common approach to ethical decision making is the 'Four principles' approach presented by Beauchamp and Childress (1). They suggest that there are four moral principles which govern the field of health care ethics, namely the principles of:

- Respect for autonomy.
- Beneficence.
- Non-maleficence.
- Distributive justice.

By considering the role and importance of each of these principles in a given situation we can hope to come to a reasonable moral decision about how to act.

Respect for autonomy

The principle of respect for autonomy recognizes the individual's right to decide upon their own destiny and to be in charge of decisions relating to themselves. In order to act autonomously an individual needs to be fully informed, competent to retain and process that information in deciding on the best course of action, and free from manipulative or coercive pressures. We cannot, therefore, respect our patients' autonomy simply by offering them a choice. We need also to ensure that they have adequate information and are not inappropriately pressured by others to choose one way rather than another.

The principle of respect for autonomy also requires that the autonomy of other members of society must be respected. There may be times when a patient's autonomous decision has to be rejected because of the effect on others. In fact, patients entering onto the LCP are unlikely to be competent to act in an autonomous manner. However, it does not follow that the principle of respect for autonomy is inapplicable in their case. They may have made advance statements when they were competent which do need to be respected. This will be discussed in more detail later.

Beneficence/non-maleficence

Beneficence is the duty to act in a way that provides benefit to others and non-maleficence is the duty not to harm. These would appear to be obvious principles to follow, both being part of our common sense understanding of morality. However, it is important to remember that neither is absolute. For example, a certain degree of harm may be necessary to provide a benefit. Frequently the opportunity to benefit a patient may be outweighed by a duty to respect one of the other principles (for example, autonomy) where a patient may decline a potentially life-saving procedure for their own individual reasons, going against what the health care professional may perceive as a benefit. Perhaps the most difficult consideration is how to decide or measure what constitutes a benefit or harm to an individual. This is likely to vary considerably from one individual to another and generally is an assessment that is best left to the patient. However in the last few days of life the patient is unlikely to be able to help with such decisions, which leaves balancing these principles to the health care professionals.

Justice

The principle of justice refers to distributive justice: the fair use and distribution of resources. (It does not refer to criminal justice in the health care context.)

At first sight, it appears to be intuitively right that resources should be divided equally between all members of society. However, criteria other than equality are also important. For example, the level of need in a particular patient and the likelihood that the health care intervention will be successful. Ensuring a fair distribution of resources seems particularly important in health care where resources are limited and the boundaries of health needs are vague. Respecting the principle of justice often results in difficult decisions with regard to the use of resources. At the end of life the right to scarce resources may seem to be less important as death is inevitable and close. Certainly expensive interventions with negligible chance of benefit should be discontinued, but some resources are usefully invested in this group. Not only do we have a moral obligation to meet the needs of symptom control and nursing care, but we must also consider the more widespread benefit during the bereavement phase of those close to the patient. A peaceful death with well-informed and supported relatives is likely to be emotionally less upsetting for all concerned.

The term 'resources' need not only refer to financial resources. Professional time is another important resource that needs to be divided equitably. Health care professionals commonly find themselves divided between a number of responsibilities and have to decide where their time is best spent. A nurse who has two patients requiring his or her help at the same time has to decide which patient to go to first. How should such decisions be made? Usually a consideration of the degree of benefit would be foremost for the health care professional in such a situation. It is easy to see how the dying patient would take second place to the patient who is likely to be cured. It is equally easy to see how such decisions can be very stressful.

Cardiopulmonary resuscitation

If "not for CPR" is to be recorded in the notes, is it necessary to discuss this with the patient and the family?

Discussion is important regarding future management, but this needs to be tailored to individual requirements and need not specifically include cardiopulmonary resuscitation (CPR). CPR is just one end of life issue out of many and this subject will be expanded on later. For patients entered on the LCP it will be futile. Discussing CPR as a separate entity only reinforces the misperception of it having life-saving properties.

Decisions relating to CPR have attracted a great deal of public attention recently. Many people have expressed fears about the withholding of a potentially life-saving procedure without prior discussion with the patient or relative. Such fears suggest that there is widespread misunderstanding of the nature and likely success of resuscitation procedures. This misperception may be perpetuated by popular television dramas portraying unrealistic success rates from CPR. It is important to recognize that success rates from CPR are low and the following factors have been associated with minimal chance of success (2):

- Metastatic cancer.
- Hypotension.

◆ Poor functional ability.

◆ Pneumonia.

What should be the approach when CPR is thought to offer no chance of success?

For patients on the LCP at the end of their lives, attempting CPR is not a life-saving procedure. It is instead an unnecessary and disturbing intervention. The evidence for this is quite clear and there can be no doubt that CPR if attempted on these patients will not prolong their lives. So in these cases CPR is to be rejected on grounds of futility. This should be clearly distinguished from a decision based on the patient's quality of life where only the patient can be in a position to judge the benefits of CPR.

The outcome from attempted CPR for LCP patients appears clear but the role of discussion when withholding CPR attempts needs more careful exploration.

It is natural for patients and families to want to be involved in such discussions and it is right that discussion should be open about all areas of care (assuming the patient is in agreement). The particular issues relating to CPR in this situation which counter this argument are as follows:

The decision of whether to attempt CPR is a clinical one and the final responsibility for the decision lies with the doctor in charge of the patient's care. Why is there a need to discuss CPR as a separate issue when it is a futile intervention with no chance of achieving the physiological aim? Especially as CPR is already wrongly considered a life-saving procedure and discussion is likely to reinforce this misperception. It seems hard to justify discussing an intervention which you have no intention of providing. As we shall go on to discuss there are many more relevant issues to raise at this time of life.

Are guidelines available to help decision making on CPR?

The fears raised by the public have resulted in a number of organizations producing guidelines which aim to allay these fears and at the same time promote good practice amongst clinicians. As a result all health care organizations should have a written policy relating to decisions about CPR. Guidance from the Association of Palliative Medicine and the National Council for Hospice and Palliative Care Services states that discussion of futile CPR with all patients is not indicated (3).

The document 'Decisions relating to cardiopulmonary resuscitation. A joint statement from the British Medical Association, the Resuscitation Council (UK), and the Royal College of Nursing' whilst recognizing that clinicians are under no obligation to provide a treatment they consider to be futile, even if the patient or family requests it, also stresses the importance of discussing CPR decisions with patients and families.

How is the discussion with the family/carer best approached?

Discussing the clinical situation regularly with patients and, with permission, families and carers is essential. Rather than focus on specific issues such as CPR however, this discussion should be more general, including their understanding of their current condition, that there are no more active treatment options, and that the focus will now be on comfort and maintaining dignity. Practical issues are also important, such as the

Ethical Decision Making in Palliative Care—Cardiopulmonary Resuscitation (CPR) for people who are terminally ill

This paper has been prepared by the National Council for Hospice and Specialist Palliative Care Services and the Association Medicine of Great Britain and Ireland. It is part of a regular update of previous guidance prepared by the two groups in August 1997 and is produced with the aim of providing guidelines for developing CPR policies.

◆ All healthcare professionals working in palliative care are committed to the value of multidisciplinary working a good communication between professionals patients and carers, especially regarding management and advanced planning at the end of life, of which cardiopulmonary resuscitation (CPR) is only one aspect.

◆ However, we recognise that units may require some guidance from the Association for Palliative Medicine and the National Council for Hospice and Specialist Palliative Care Services in developing their approach and policies regarding CPR. This is particularly so in the light of the recent document from the BMA, Royal College of Nursing, Resuscitation Council (UK) – Decisions relating to Cardiopulmonary Resuscitation, The Human Rights Act 1998 (implemented October 2000) and the Health Service Circular reference no 2000/028.

◆ As we understand the Human Rights Act (Article 2), the right to life does not entail the right to treatment that is judged by a clinician to be very unlikely to achieve its physiological aim of prolonging life. No doctor can be required to deliver a treatment which he or she believes is not clinically justifiable.

◆ We reaffirm that there is no ethical obligation to discuss CPR with those palliative care patients, for whom such treatment, following assessment, is judged to be futile. If however, the likely outcome of a CPR intervention is uncertain, anticipatory decisions, either to implement or withhold CPR should be sensitively explored with appropriate individual patients.

◆ In many specialist palliative care units it is possible to provide only basic CPR for patients, visitors and staff. Basic CPR involves artificial ventilation using either a mask- or mouth-to-mouth techniques along with compression of the chest wall to maintain circulation.

◆ There is now a requirement for all units to ensure that policies regarding CPR are in place and that this information is available to patients. We would suggest that written information given to patients should contain a general statement on the principles by which treatment decisions are made in palliative care and an explanation of the facilities that the unit can provide for CPR on site.

Reproduced with the kind permission of the National Council for Hospices and Specialist Palliative Care

need to arrange time off from work, contacting members of the family or friends, etc. The emphasis should be on what is in the patient's best interest rather than interventions that will not offer any benefit. As a result of such discussion there would be little benefit in specifically discussing attempted CPR because all parties are informed of the stage of the illness and the future possibilities. Such discussions should always be recorded in the notes. Apart from the obvious legal reasons for this it also informs other members of the team of the situation and views of key individuals.

What if families or friends ask about CPR?

Families may wish to raise the issue of CPR specifically. It is useful to begin such discussion by gaining an understanding of their perceptions of CPR and what they hope it would achieve. The harm caused by CPR in terms of lack of dignity and possible pain and discomfort to the patient with no resulting life prolongation are the key issues to raise. The moral justification rests on these issues.

Should families or friends be asked to make CPR decisions?

Asking families or friends to make decisions about attempting futile CPR can be harmful. Without the clinical knowledge families may feel they have denied the patient a life-saving procedure, perhaps causing their death. This misperception can be a source of great anxiety and may make the bereavement process more difficult.

Issues of hydration

If the patient is no longer taking fluids by mouth, is it ethical not to hydrate them with intravenous or subcutaneous fluids?

In this situation it is usually in the patient's best interests not to receive artificial hydration and therefore this is morally justified.

The key issue is to distinguish a patient who is dying from their disease from one who is dying because they are unable to maintain their hydration. If the patient is not in the dying phase, then artificial hydration may well be indicated. A patient who is confused, with infection or metabolic disturbance such as hypercalcaemia, may gain significant benefit from rehydration. Similarly a patient with a physical obstruction, such as carcinoma of the oesophagus, may need artificial hydration until the situation can be resolved. Patients coming onto the LCP should have had such conditions excluded.

For the patient in the dying phase the moral decision rests on the benefits and harms of artificial hydration. A patient entering the dying phase is often only able to take sips of fluid and as they approach death they are unlikely to be taking anything by mouth. This appears to be a natural physiological process and experience in palliative care suggests patients die quite peacefully and comfortably without the use of artificial hydration. Studies support this by demonstrating that there are few biochemical disturbances indicating dehydration at the end of life (4). It is likely that symptoms associated with dry mouth are caused more by medication and mouth breathing than by lack of fluid. Appropriate mouth care would be the most effective way to counter this symptom.

There are a number of potential risks or harms from artificial hydration including: excess respiratory secretions, oedema, and site problems from the intravenous or subcutaneous infusions. The necessary equipment may interfere with contact between the patient and families at a very emotionally sensitive time.

The suggested benefits of artificial hydration include helping symptoms of dry mouth, thirst, headache, confusion, and exhaustion. Unfortunately there is no strong evidence for either point of view as comparative studies are not possible. For families, the provision of hydration may seem an essential part of human existence and quite understandably it may cause distress, when it is withheld. The instinct to provide fluid and nutrition to a person who is poorly is very basic, and perhaps this is one of the few areas that families may feel able to influence. Some health care professionals may hold the same view. It is important to consider all these aspects and listen carefully to the worries which are expressed. The accepted practice in palliative care in the United Kingdom is that the harm caused by hydration once the patient enters the dying phase is greater than any benefit. Hydration is not a life-prolonging procedure, neither is the lack of hydration the cause of death of the patient. The patient is dying from their underlying disease and the presence or absence of artificial hydration will not influence this. Guidance from the Association of Palliative Medicine and the National Council for Hospice and Palliative Care Services states that an individual approach to each case is advisable when considering artificial hydration (5).

The emotional upset caused to a family from withholding artificial nutrition may outweigh the suggested benefit to the patient. It is important in these situations to understand their ideas, concerns, and expectations. Usually a discussion of the harm of artificial hydration leaves families fairly contented. However, if strong concerns remain, a trial of artificial hydration may help to reassure them that such an intervention will not benefit their relative.

If the patient is no longer taking fluids by mouth, is it ethical to discontinue artificial hydration in the dying phase?

To discontinue artificial hydration in this situation is entirely justifiable. The answer to the previous question addresses how the harms of artificial hydration outweigh any potential benefits and therefore why usual practice is not to commence this intervention.

Is the situation different if the patient already has an infusion running—should this be stopped?

Intuitively it seems that to take something away is harder to justify than not commencing the intervention in the first place. The Acts/Omissions Doctrine (AOD) states that there is a moral difference between acting and omitting to act, even where the outcomes are identical. In this situation acting to withdraw hydration already in progress would be, according to the AOD, harder to justify than failing to initiate it. However, closer examination of the principles involved shows that withdrawing and withholding a treatment are often morally equivalent, so it's hard to see how to justify the Acts/Omissions Doctrine.

National Hospice Council for Hospice and Specialist Palliative Care Services Ethical Decision Making in Palliative Care—Artificial Hydration for people who are terminally ill

This paper has been prepared by a Joint Working Party between the National Hospice Council for Hospice and Specialist Palliative Care Services and the Ethics Committee for the Association of Palliative Medicine for Great Britain and Ireland.

The paper is concerned with artificial hydration by naso-gastric tube, gastrostomy, or subcutaneous or intravenous drip. It should be noted that good practice suggests decisions regarding artificial hydration should involve a multidisciplinary team, the patient, and relatives and carers, but that the senior doctor has ultimate responsibility for the decision. However, a competent patient has the right to refuse artificial hydration, even if it may be considered of clinical benefit. Incompetent patients retain this right through a valid advance refusal.

1. A blanket policy of artificial hydration, or of no artificial hydration, is ethically indefensible.

2. Towards death, a person's desire for food and drink lessens. Study evidence is limited but suggests that artificial hydration in imminently dying patients influences neither survival nor symptom control. As such it may constitute an unnecessary intrusion.

3. Thirst or dry mouth in people who are terminally ill may frequently be caused by medication. In such circumstances artificial hydration is unlikely to alleviate the symptom. Good mouth care and reassessment of medication become the most appropriate interventions.

4. Appropriate palliative care will involve consideration of the option of artificial hydration, where dehydration results from a potentially correctable cause (e.g. over-treatment with diuretics and sedation, recurrent vomiting, diarrhoea and hyper-calcaemia).

5. It is a responsibility of the clinical team to make assessments concerning the relevance of hydration to the experience of individual patients. The appropriateness of artificial hydration should be judged on a day-to-day basis, weighing up the potential harms and benefits. The practicalities of appropriate provision will vary according to setting, but good practice will require that patients needing artificial hydration are transferred to a unit equipped to provide such care.

6. Relatives at the bedside of dying patients frequently express concern about lack of fluid or nutrient intake. Health care professionals may not subordinate the interests of patients to the anxieties of relatives but should, nevertheless, strive to address those anxieties.

The appropriateness of artificial hydration continues to depend on regular assessment of the likely benefits and burdens of such intervention.

Reproduced with the kind permission of the National Council for Hospices and Specialist Palliative Care

If we consider how the four principles apply to this situation, the essence of this decision remains the benefit against harm ratio. The arguments remain the same as in the previous section; the previous presence of hydration does not influence them. In addition, it is not the act or the omission that is important. The key aspect is the intention of the health care professional. In withdrawing artificial hydration the health care professional intends to improve the overall comfort of the patient and to try to prevent any harm. This is just the same as the intention of the health care professional who decides not to start hydration in a similar situation.

Foreshortening life/euthanasia

If a patient is dying and is given medication to relieve symptoms, e.g. subcutaneous diamorphine for pain, and then dies a few minutes later, is this euthanasia?

The health care professional in this situation is not performing euthanasia.

Euthanasia is defined as the intentional bringing about of the death of a patient, either by killing him/her or by allowing him/her to die, for the patient's own sake. Euthanasia or physician-assisted suicide (PAS) remain illegal in the UK, although there is greater acceptance of this practice in some other countries.

It is important to distinguish this from other decisions made at the end of life, where death may result but is not the *intention* of the person taking the action. The health care professional in this situation cannot be performing euthanasia because their intention is not to cause the patient's death but to improve their comfort. Any risk of shortening the patient's life may be justified under the doctrine of double effect (DDE).

The DDE states that a bad effect such as a patient's death may be permissible if it is not intended and occurs as a side-effect of a beneficial action. In order to justify this position four criteria have to be met (6):

(a) The intended end, in this case the relief of pain, must be a good one.

(b) The bad effect, the patient's death, may be foreseen but must not be intended.

(c) The bad effect must not be the means of bringing about the good effect, so the death of the patient cannot be the method by which the pain is relieved.

(d) The good effect must on balance outweigh the bad effect, so for a patient in the dying phase the risk of shortening life for the benefit of comfort is considerably less than in an otherwise healthy individual.

In the United Kingdom the DDE has been recognized in law in the following circumstances:

(a) The patient must be terminally ill so that it is the illness and not the medication that causes death.

(b) The treatment must be right and proper as accepted by a responsible body of medical opinion.

(c) The motivation for the treatment must be to relieve suffering.

In practice, although health care professionals often worry about the safety of opioids and sedatives in this group of patients, experience suggests that this is more of a theoretical concern than a real one.

A study looking at 238 consecutive deaths at a large palliative care unit showed the DDE was rarely if ever used to justify opioid use in dying patients (7). When opioids are used appropriately to control symptoms there is little need to rapidly increase doses and no apparent decrease in survival. The study suggests that if a health care professional was having to double doses of opioids or felt they had to implement the DDE to justify their actions this should indicate a need for specialist palliative care advice.

Nonetheless health care professionals are often left with a feeling that it was their action in giving or prescribing the last injection that caused the death. This is a feeling that may be uncomfortable for some. In reality it is hard to know for sure whether it is the injection that caused the death of the patient as it must be remembered that symptoms worsen towards the end of life and increased use of symptomatic treatments is therefore necessary. Death may well have occurred at that time even without intervention.

Is the use of sedation justified in the same way?

Morally and legally the use of sedatives is justified in the same manner. The use of opioids is quite specific for pain or dyspnoea, but the possible role for sedatives is far broader including any symptom or psychological issue that causes distress and cannot be resolved in other ways. Estimates vary but sedation is used to relieve unendurable symptoms in about 15–36% of patients in some palliative care units (8). This may cause anxiety as the treatment is less specific, more open to abuse, and seems intuitively more difficult to justify. However, the principles previously discussed apply similarly here. An agitated, anxious, confused, or breathless dying patient causes distress not only to themselves but all those watching. The use of sedatives in this situation is likely to be the only way to offer relief and is generally considered as essential to good symptom control at the end of life. A number of studies have indicated no difference in survival with appropriate use of sedation.

If the multidisciplinary team decide that a patient is in the dying phase, but the relatives want all active treatment to be continued, how should the views of the relatives influence the decision making of the multidisciplinary team?

The ultimate responsibility for treatment decisions lies with the patient and the doctor in charge of their care. A doctor cannot treat a competent patient against their will, but neither can they be forced to provide a treatment that has no benefit to the patient. The approach to this situation usually starts with a decision as to whether the patient is competent. Patients in the dying phase are likely to be only semi-conscious and therefore unable to make decisions such as these. The clinician in charge of their care should then make decisions based on what he or she feels is in the best interests of the patient. This is based not only on clinical factors but also on their prior knowledge of the patient's wishes and any advance statements they may have made. It is good practice to discuss these factors with the multidisciplinary team to achieve a consensus and also to ensure as far as possible all the relevant information has been gathered.

If we apply the 'four principles' approach to this situation there is little role for respect for autonomy, unless the patient has made an advance directive, because the patient is unlikely to be competent to make informed choices. A decision to avoid unnecessary active treatment is supported by a duty to act beneficently towards the patient and avoid unnecessary harm. A duty to distribute resources justly suggests we should not initiate such treatment.

It is also good practice to discuss issues with those close to the patient and to keep them informed of the situation when a patient is dying. Such discussions may help the health care professional to understand what the patient themselves would have wanted at this time and so reach the most appropriate conclusions. Relatives may not hold the same views as the patient, and if asked to make a decision the answer is likely to be what they would want for themselves or to use the patient's 'off the cuff' remarks as a basis for the decision. Relatives may not wish themselves to be seen as the person responsible for withdrawing treatments and so may be more proactive. Conflicts within families are common and will impair balanced decision making. At the extreme there may be concerns regarding the motives behind the making of certain requests. Relatives are unable to insist on interventions or treatment that a multidisciplinary team do not feel is in the patient's best interests and this position is recognized in law. However, a good understanding of the situation and a trusting relationship with the multidisciplinary team is important for the families' emotional well being and the bereavement process that is to follow.

Good communication in these situations is of key importance. Providing regular updates on the situation and taking time to pass on decisions, may well prevent difficulties at a later stage. Blunt declarations that the decision is not theirs to make, or failure to discuss the relatives' suggestions is unhelpful and potentially damaging. A careful exploration of why they are requesting active treatment and their understanding of their relative's condition, usually helps to resolve most difficulties.

Advanced directives

How should an advance directive affect the care of a dying patient?

Advance directives or statements should be recognized as a valid means by which patients can influence the treatments they receive when they are no longer competent to make decisions. Patients cannot insist on additional treatments. This remains the decision of the medical team. However, they can refuse interventions other than basic care such as washing or pain relief. A recent study showed the benefit of discussing advance statements with patients and suggests that such discussions could be incorporated into routine history taking (9).

There is recognition in law for such statements although they offer a number of benefits in resolving difficult end of life issues for the health care professional and help to relieve the family and carers from what they might perceive as an unwanted responsibility for advising over treatment decisions. They enable health care professionals to show respect for the principle of autonomy and to know what the patient would have perceived as being in their best interests, a decision clinicians can sometimes find difficult.

When presented with an advance directive it is important for health care professionals to clarify whether the patient was competent at the time of making the statement and whether they foresaw the situation they now find themselves in. The date of making the directive may also be relevant, as new developments may have occurred since the time of making the statement, which could alter the choices they would have made. A specific format is not required and advance directives can be either written or oral. A well prepared directive offers greater reassurance to the health care professional, especially if the contents go against medical advice. A number of organizations have prepared standard formats which may be useful. The wording of the statement needs to strike a balance between being specific enough to relate to the situation faced and yet broad enough to cover all scenarios that may be encountered. Statements should be regularly reviewed and need to be readily accessible. Relatives or carers need to know of their existence and ideally be comfortable with their contents.

Advance directives offer the opportunity for treatment decisions at the end of life to be in keeping with the patient's wishes. In their preparation and activation they demonstrate a willingness from the medical profession to listen to patients' wishes. It is possible that their use may increase over the next few years and they are likely to become an increasingly important factor in making end of life decisions.

References

1. Beauchamp, T. L. and Childress, J. F. (1994). *Principles of biomedical ethics*. Oxford University Press, New York.
2. Beddel, S. E., Delbanco, T. L., Cook, F. E., and Epstein, F. H. (1983). Survival after CPR in the hospital. *N. Engl. J. Med.*, 309, 569–75.
3. Joint Working Party between the National Council for Hospice and Specialist Palliative Care Services and the Ethics Committee of the Association for Palliative Medicine of Great Britain and Ireland. (2002). *Ethical decision making: Cardiopulmonary resuscitation (CPR) for people who are terminally ill*. National Council for Hospital and Specialist Palliative Care Services.
4. Ellershaw, J. E., Sutcliffe, J. M., and Saunders, C. M. (1995). Dehydration and the dying patient. *J. Pain Symptom Manage.*, 10(3), 192–7.
5. Joint Working Party between the National Council for Hospice and Specialist Palliative Care Services and the Ethics Committee of the Association for Palliative Medicine of Great Britain and Ireland. (1997). Ethical decision making in palliative care: Artificial hydration for people who are terminally ill. *J. Eur. Assoc. Palliat. Care*, 4(4), 124.
6. Thorns, A. (1998). A review of the doctrine of double effect. *Eur. J. Palliat. Care*, 5(4), 117–20.
7. Thorns, A. R. and Sykes, N. P. (2000). Opioid use in the last week of life and the implications for end of life decision-making. *Lancet*, 356, 398–9.
8. Fainsinger, R. L., Waller, A., Bercovici, M., Bengston, K., Landman, W., Hosking, M., et al. (2000). A multicentre international study of sedation for uncontrolled symptoms in terminally ill patients. *Palliat. Med.*, 14(4), 257–65.
9. Sayers, G. M., Barratt, D., Gothard, C., Onnie, C., Perera, S., and Schulman, D. (2001). The value of taking an 'ethics history'. *J. Med. Ethics*, 27, 114–17.

Chapter 5

Communication in care of the dying

Susie Wilkinson and Carole Mula

Introduction

A major component of the delivery of the Liverpool Integrated Care Pathway for the Dying Patient (LCP) is communication. Communication has been defined in a variety of ways. For the purpose of this chapter communication is defined as "an interchange of thoughts, feelings and opinions among individuals. Verbal communication is effective when it satisfies basic desires for recognition, participation, and self-realisation by direct personal contact between persons" (1).

Whether communication is verbal or non-verbal it occurs during every encounter between a nurse and a patient. Research evidence suggests individuals do not become effective communicators from experience alone. It is also necessary to learn and understand certain skills and knowledge, and explore personal and societal attitudes (2, 3).

There is a general assumption that effective communication is achieved when open two-way communication takes place, and patients are informed about the nature of their illness and treatment and are encouraged to express their anxieties and emotions. This view assumes that open communication, full information about a disease and its prognosis, has benefits for all patients.

In reality though the issue is much more complex and the key for all health professionals is to be able to tailor their communication to the patients' communication and information needs. In palliative care the challenges are even greater than usual because of the expectation that health professionals will be able to discuss and cope with death and loss (4).

The importance of supportive communication was poignantly highlighted by an American oncology nurse dying of breast cancer. Days before her death she completed a paper, delivered posthumously by her husband as the 12th recipient of the Mara Morgensen Flaherty Memorial lecture at the Oncology Nursing Society Congress. Bushkin wrote, "There are so many questions, concerns and problems to face in the lightening ball mirror. To overcome the sense of powerlessness the traveller (i.e. patient) runs through a maze seeking someone who might actually listen to their pleas for help, someone who actually knows that the traveller is there. The question of being heard and having one's questions answered is a perpetual source of frustration. In the absence of recognition the traveller feels alone and at the mercy of those who do not hear" (5).

Effective communication is central to good patient care. Health professionals' psychosocial skills have been shown to determine patients' satisfaction, compliance, and health outcomes, even to the extent that if health professionals explore patients' concerns and feelings even when their concerns cannot be resolved a significant fall in patient anxiety levels is noted (6).

Patients however continue to be dissatisfied with health care and this is in part related to ineffective communication and poor attitudes between patients, their families, and health professionals (7–10). Communication difficulties are found to be particularly problematic when a patient faces a terminal illness as identified by the Health Ombudsman, "I find it hard to comprehend failure by members of the caring professions to communicate adequately with patients, particularly those who are terminally ill" (11).

There is however good evidence that communication skills can be taught (12–16). The chapter therefore proposes to raise awareness of the communication skills necessary to promote the principles of high quality care which is the aim of the LCP. As Thorns and Garrard emphasized (Chapter 4), good communication skills are vital for effectively communicating any moral decisions made to patients or their families. The chapter will therefore address the communication skills required to handle the many difficult situations that frequently arise when caring for dying patients.

What are the skills that facilitate communication?

Patients are more likely to disclose their concerns to those professionals who demonstrate that they are prepared to listen and are open to discussion (17). This involves the use of verbal and non-verbal communication skills which facilitate the patient and their relatives to discuss their worries or concerns.

Non-verbal communication plays a large part in portraying how patients feel. Health professionals' non-verbal behaviours often demonstrate to patients a commitment to listening to their concerns. The importance of adopting good non-verbal behaviours cannot be over-emphasized and are briefly described in Table 5.1.

In caring for dying patients, there are vital verbal skills to be adopted. Verbal communication can be divided into two parts; the language, i.e. the actual words used, paralanguage, i.e. how it is said, for example, the tone of voice, volume, pitch, clarity, and rate.

Table 5.2 describes the main verbal skills with examples that facilitate good communication. However some behaviours that often are thought by health professionals to be facilitating for patients, in fact hinder communication and can prevent patients and relatives disclosing their concerns.

Blocking tactics that can hinder communication

Blocking tactics were first noted by Quint (18) who observed health professionals interacting with patients with breast cancer. Over twenty years later Wilkinson (3) described a more comprehensive account of the behaviours that were still being used to block communication. Most of the nurses involved in the study were unaware that the behaviours they were using hindered communication.

These behaviours are:

(a) **Normalizing**: Automatic placatory comments that convey either a lack of understanding from the patient's point of view, or that the patient's experiences are not unique or important. These comments simply shift the focus away from the patient. e.g. " ... everyone feels frightened of dying ...." .

Table 5.1 Adoptive behaviours of professionals, patients, and relatives

Personal space	Area around the body, which, if intruded by some people, leaves one feeling uncomfortable. Professionals need to sit down squarely in relation to the patient to allow all aspects of communication to be seen; paralinguistic, such as sighs, grunts, and non-verbal bodily communication. Professionals need to lean towards the patient to encourage them and make them feel more understood.
Facial expressions	Display emotions, which may conflict or support the spoken word, i.e. nodding, agreeing or disagreeing, frown lines, position of the eye brows and eye lids, size of pupils.
Eye contact	Important in building satisfying relationships; should be reasonably sustained. Ratio of contact professional: patient = 1 : 1. Avoidance can signal discomfort or disinterest
Posture	Demonstrates attitudes, emotions, and mood; supports or conflicts the spoken word. Open position to be adopted in relation to the patient.
	A 'closed' position, such as crossing both arms and legs, conveys defensive feeling.
Gestures	Illustrates speech, expresses emotions, i.e. raising a finger, increased hand movements indicating anxiety, minimal hand movements indicating depression.
Touching	Helps develop a caring relationship; expresses emotion. Dying patients often feel the need for physical contact with carers; holding hands provides physical expression to the personal relationship.

(b) **False or premature reassurance:** Remarks and comments made to the patient which provide a false or premature sense of reassurance and are more positive than the situation warrants.
e.g. "… you won't have any pain because we will give you pain killers…".

(c) **Inappropriate advice:** Advice which encourages a decision to be made by the patient by imposing one's own opinions and solutions, as opposed to assisting the patient with exploration of ways of arriving at a conclusion.
e.g. (*patient*) "…I don't know whether to take this sedative…".
(*professional*) "Well I would if it was me."

(d) **Leading questions:** A question is asked in such a way as to predetermine a particular response from a patient.
e.g. "You are looking fine, you must be feeling fine?"

(e) **Closed questions:** Type of question that can restrict the range of possible responses from a patient, encouraging a monosyllabic 'yes' or 'no' as opposed to inviting discussion or expression of feeling.
e.g. "Any problems with your sleep?" as opposed to "How are you sleeping?"

Table 5.2 Verbal skills

Listening	An active skill that requires great concentration if the patient's cues are to be addressed.	
Silences	Allows both parties to think and assimilate what has been said.	
Acknowledgement	Utterances that indicate the patient is being heard and taken note of.	*Mmmh, uuh, yes.*
Encouragement	More active than acknowledgement. Importance in the maintenance of interaction. Actively showing interest and understanding, encourages the patient to continue.	*Really, that is interesting, please do go on.*
Picking up cues	Patients drop hints or cues of problems. The skill lies in being able to pick up on these.	*Q: How are you today? A: I'm fine really, it's the family that have been upsetting me. The cue is highlighted.*
Reflection	Encourages discussion around a problem raised and in depth/ further analysis.	*The family have been upsetting you, in what way have they been upsetting you?*
Open questioning	Provide room for patients to express themselves. Elicit feelings.	*How do you feel today? How have you been sleeping?*
Clarification	Questions to ensure the patient's meaning is understood. Enables more detailed information on problems to emerge.	*Q: I'm feeling non-plussed A: What do you mean by that? Or Q: That will be it. A: What exactly do you mean by that will be it?*
Empathy	Statements which demonstrate understanding from the patients' point of view. Encourage the patient to go into more depth.	*It sounds as if things have been very hard for you lately. Or From what you have said, I get the feeling that you have been feeling very low.*
Confrontation/ challenge	Questions or statements that challenge discrepancies in what patients say.	*You've said you are feeling fine and have no worries, but you have just said that you are feeling anxious. Can you tell me a bit more about this?*
Information giving	Patients should only be given required information. Assessment of this informational needs should be done prior to release of information. Patients are only able to retain small amounts of data at a time; this needs to be given slowly, without jargon or technical terms.	

(f) **Multiple questioning:** Questions can be asked in a confusing torrent without pausing for a reply to each.
e.g. "How do you feel? Have you any pain? Did you sleep well?"

(g) **Passing the buck:** Deflecting the patient to another colleague when asked a specific and uncomfortable question.
e.g. "Ask the doctor about this when you next see him."

(h) **Asking for an explanation:** Analysis is passed back to the patient by asking for an explanation of feelings or actions, sometimes with an intimidating and stark 'why'?
e.g. (*patient*) "I didn't sleep last night."
(*professional*) "Why didn't you sleep?"

(i) **Approving/agreeing:** Remarks and opinions can shift the focus to the professionals' own feelings and values. This imposes upon and restricts the patients' own free expression.
e.g. (*patient*) "My family have been worrying me."
(*professional*) "I think you need to stop worrying about your family and concentrate on getting better."

(j) **Defensive behaviours:** When a patient becomes angry or worried, excuses are made rather than allowing the patient to explore and express his feelings and opinions.
e.g. (*patient*) "I'm really worried about dying."
(*professional*) "Oh the chaplain is really good, he is the expert."

(k) **Shifting the focus to relatives:** In discussions with the patient, focus can be shifted from his problems to the relative and thus emphasis is removed from how the patient feels, to how his relatives feel or think.
e.g. (*patient*) "I think I'm going to find it hard going into the hospice."
(*professional*) "What does your wife think about it?"

(l) **Selective attention to cues:** When cues or questions are raised, a response is selected to address the physical rather than the emotional aspects.
e.g. (*patient*) "My pain has gone, but I'm feeling very low."
(*professional*) "I'm pleased your pain has gone."

(m) **Jollying along:** Some bright and cheerful placatory remarks or comments are merely glossing over real issues in the hope that the patient will feel better. These in fact make the patient feel uneasy in stating their true feelings.
e.g. "Don't look so glum! It's a gorgeous day outside. Give me a smile."

(n) **Irrelevant chit chat:** Personal irrelevant chit chat removes the focus of the interaction from the patient and their concerns, back to the professional.

The reason for describing these behaviours is because many health professionals have adopted them by habit without realizing the effects. This is not to say they should never be used. There are situations when they are used as protection for our own emotional stability in an often very stressful area of care. However in order to help patients, their use should be minimized.

Once the basic communication skills have been mastered they need to be put into action to address the situations that arise when patients commence the LCP.

Are the patient and their family aware of the patient's deteriorating condition?

Interviewing and assessment skills form the basis of all communication interaction (19). The uniqueness of each patient can only be recognized by carrying out a comprehensive assessment which addresses the patient's agenda (19). Some health professionals undervalue the role of an assessment and see it merely as a form filling exercise (20). Assessment however is possibly the most vital part of care as without an accurate assessment it is not possible to plan good quality individualized care. There are nine key areas of assessment (Table 5.3) which amount to a comprehensive assessment of a patient, however the assessment most appropriate for establishing the patients insight into their condition is the assessment of the patients awareness of their diagnosis.

Patient's awareness of diagnosis

To assess the patient's insight of their diagnosis, the discussion needs to be carefully organized in terms of setting adequate time aside, agreeing the venue, and giving the patient the option to have a relative(s) present if he wishes who may provide valuable support.

The venue should be a quiet and private setting away from interruptions and distractions such as telephone calls, bleeps, and uninvited visitors. This is to ensure privacy for the patient and relatives to encourage an open dialogue. However, it is recognized that in some care settings (such as a main ward within a hospital), it is sometimes difficult to provide privacy. In such cases, make the situation as private as possible by screening an area off and informing staff of the intended discussions. The amount and level of detailed information about the patient's diagnosis and prognosis needs to be guided by both verbal and non-verbal cues from the patient.

To gain the patient's confidence and trust, let the patient tell their story and establish their understanding for admission not just what the doctor has said.

◆ *Can you tell me what you understand about your illness?*
◆ *How did you feel when the doctor told you about your illness?*
◆ *How do you feel things are going for you just now?*
◆ *What thoughts have you had about your illness?*

Table 5.3 Key areas of patient assessment

Introduction to assessment.
Patient's understanding of admission.
Patient's awareness of diagnosis.
Patient's history of present illness.
Patient's history of previous illness.
Physical assessment.
Social assessment.
Psychological assessment.
Closure of assessment.

♦ *What would you like to know about your illness that might help you gain a better understanding about your diagnosis?*

Establish with whom the patient has a meaningful relationship and the extent of support from the relationship.

♦ *How is your family coping with your illness?*

♦ *Which family member would you like me to talk with?*

Establish the patient's present mood state, in terms of how the illness is affecting them. Pick up on any cues as to how the patient has been feeling in terms of anxiety and depression.

♦ *What has been the most difficult part of this illness?*

♦ *What is the worst thing that could happen?*

♦ *Is there anything in particular that makes you feel frightened?*

Handling difficult questions

Some patients in the final stages of their life are aware of the significance of certain symptoms, such as increasing weakness and weight loss that confirms the fact that death is approaching and that they are dying, and often pose questions like, "Am I dying?" or "I'm not going to get better am I?" Figure 5.1 outlines a structure of a possible way to handle such difficult questions.

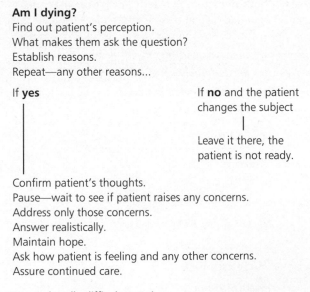

Am I dying?
Find out patient's perception.
What makes them ask the question?
Establish reasons.
Repeat—any other reasons...

If **yes**

If **no** and the patient
changes the subject

Leave it there, the
patient is not ready.

Confirm patient's thoughts.
Pause—wait to see if patient raises any concerns.
Address only those concerns.
Answer realistically.
Maintain hope.
Ask how patient is feeling and any other concerns.
Assure continued care.

Figure 5.1 How to handle difficult questions.

What has Happened for the patient to ask the question?

The patient obviously has been thinking about the issue, otherwise they would not have asked the question. It is therefore necessary to explore the patient's thought processes, guiding them with a question such as, "I'm happy to talk to you about the question you have asked but it would just help me if you could tell me what, if anything, has prompted you to ask me this question today?" The patient may respond that for one or two reasons they feel that they are not getting better.

Checking readiness for receiving bad news

Whether the patient is likely to cope psychologically with bad news can sometimes be judged by first establishing whether the patient is ready to receive confirmation of their own thoughts. Some patients ask a question and then wish that they had not, particularly if they perceive the news will be bad. To guard against this it is sometimes a good idea to give the patient a second chance by asking them, "You've given me one or two reasons why you feel that you are not getting any better, or you feel that you are dying, are there any other reasons?" The patient now has two options. They can either say that there are some additional reasons for feeling they are deteriorating or dying, or they can simply change the subject, thus demonstrating that they are not actually ready to receive bad news at that point in time.

Confirming bad news

If the patient gives other reasons as to why they feel they are dying, this is a good indication that they are aware of their situation. In this instance there is only one path open, to confirm to the patient that their thoughts are correct. For example, "It appears from what you've said that you feel that you are dying and yes, I'm afraid I think your thoughts are correct, and you may well die from this illness." A typical reaction from health professionals on having broken bad news is a desire to make the situation better for the patient by giving information on how symptoms for example can be controlled. This can result in actually giving reassurance for symptoms that the patient may not have thought about. It is therefore necessary to wait until the patient raises their concerns or worries, and then address those concerns alone. Common fears and concerns are listed in Table 5.4.

Table 5.4 Common fears and concerns for some dying patients

Debility.
Loss of independence.
The thought of the dying process.
Possible loss of control.
Uncontrolled pain.
Fighting for breath.
The moment of death.
How death will occur.
What happens after death.
Unfinished business.

Dealing with patients questions realistically

Answer patients questions realistically. If the patient asks if they will experience any pain, rather than saying, "Oh, no, you won't have any pain, we will look after that", it is far better to go through with the patient the different methods of controlling pain, and reassure the patient that you will do your best and hopefully they will not be in pain.

This kind of response is the one that helps to maintain patients' hope. By indicating that while it may not be possible to effect the outcome of their situation, there is still a great deal of care that can be given to alleviate distressing symptoms. Once concerns raised have been addressed, ascertain how the patient is feeling and if they have any other concerns they would like to discuss. If there are no concerns at that present moment in time, convey to the patient that any future concerns can be discussed at a later date.

Communicating with relatives

As patients deteriorate, relatives too need the opportunity to ask questions about the significance of the patient's deterioration and be given appropriate explanations. This reinforces that the patient has reached the terminal phase where death is imminent. At this time it is also important to identify how the family wish to be informed about the patient's death. For example, who should be contacted should a further deterioration occur. For many relatives, being present at the time of death is very important. It is therefore necessary to establish at what stage the family would like to be called in should the patient's condition deteriorate and where and when they wish to be contacted, i.e. night or day or at work.

Some relatives may wish to stay overnight with the patient and, depending on the conditions within the organization, this will determine whether it is possible or not.

It is common for relatives who stay overnight with the patient to feel a compulsion to stay by the patient's bedside constantly. Thus, they become anxious about leaving and often need encouragement from staff to take some time out.

Many dying patients, increasingly dependent upon professionals and relatives, convey feelings of extreme fatigue, and although they may wish for relatives to be present, they feel a dilemma of being over-visited but yet are unable to express their feelings without being insensitive to the needs of their family.

Thus, sensitive communications, often on behalf of the patient, should take place and agreements reached to set limits on the number and frequency of agreed visitors. One way forward may be the suggestion of a visiting rota to enable both patient and visitors to get some rest.

If the relatives are with the patient when they die, many are often not aware death has actually occurred. Therefore they need to be taken aside and informed sensitively and with empathy that the patient has died. The words death and died should always be used as this is highlighted as one of the goals of the LCP. Euphemisms such as passed away, passed on should not be used as these just reinforce the taboo of talking about death and dying that exists in modern society. A recent anecdotal example illustrates how if the word death or dying is not used relatives can be confused. A patient following a road traffic accident was admitted to A&E. Resuscitation was taking place when the relatives arrived and this was explained to the relatives. When resuscitation failed the doctor informed the relatives who were in a state of shock that they were sorry they had 'lost him'. The relatives, not realizing the patient had died went for a cup of tea and returned an hour later to ask if the patient had been found. This very unfortunate incident clearly reinforces how important it is to use the correct words when communicating with relatives.

Communicating with families who want to protect patients from the truth

Many relatives wish to protect their loved ones from receiving bad news, and ask health professionals not to disclose bad news. To overcome this situation it is necessary to gain the relatives' confidence so that they do not think the patient would be unilaterally approached and told that they are dying. One way of coping with this situation is shown in Figure 5.2. It is vital initially to accept what the relative has requested by saying "I can entirely agree with what you are saying, but can I ask you though how you are?", and find out how the relative feels they are coping, and communicating with their loved one. This often highlights that relatives are under considerable strain. Keeping the truth from the patient is stressful. It is sometimes appropriate to actually highlight that collusion can strain a relationship.

Once the relatives' feelings have been explored, the reasons for them not wanting to be truthful with the patient need to be discussed. Whatever the reason it is important that these reasons are supported. The next step is to ask the relative whether the patient has in fact asked any questions about their illness. In most cases the patient will have asked some questions. It is therefore vital to suggest that because the patient has asked some questions it indicates that they may have some idea of their true condition.

The relative still needs reassurance that the patient's condition will not just be divulged to them, but it needs to be pointed out that, as the health professional looking after them, you will need to find out how the patient is feeling and whether they have any concerns or worries to discuss. It is also important to 'flag up' to the relative that, should in the course of discussions the patient disclose that they know that they

* Focus on relatives':
    * feelings
    * reasons for not being truthful
    * strain on relationship
* Support reasons
* Assess patients' questions to relatives
* Suggest window on knowledge
* Ask for permission to assess relatives
* Reassure no telling
* Confirmation if necessary

Figure 5.2 Collusion.

are dying and are able to substantiate their reasons as to why they think they are dying, it would only be fair and ethical to confirm the patient's own assessment of the situation. If the patient does disclose that they are aware of their true condition, it is then necessary to make contact with the family and inform them that whilst talking to the patient they raised concerns about their weight loss and whether that meant they were dying, and that you responded to this question by confirming to the patient that they were correct in their belief. Frequently relatives are concerned that the patient will 'fall apart' or be very distressed. It is therefore important to stress to the relatives (if appropriate) that the patient was naturally upset but was relieved that they now know. In some cases this serves to enable the patient and their family to share feelings at a very difficult time.

Handling feelings and emotions

Often when patients or relatives have been told bad news they experience emotions such as anger and anxiety. A strategy for handling feelings and emotions is shown in Figure 5.3.

If people become very distressed and cry, acknowledge that they are upset by saying, for example, "I can see that you are really upset by what I have just told you and I would like you to explain just how upset you feel and if there are any specific issues or feelings that you would like to share." This kind of approach usually facilitates the patient to actually talk about their upset.

It is then important to accept what the patient says empathetically. Summarize how they feel, for example, "You sound as if you are upset because…, and I understand that you are upset." Empathy facilitates the patient to discuss their distress. Empathy is a skill that is not widely used but it offers patients very gently an opportunity to talk (3). Sometimes patients prefer not to discuss their distress and they will say so and their decision must be respected. Empathy is the ability to perceive the meaning and feelings of another person and communicate that feeling to the other person (21). Kalilsch (22) believes empathy is the ability to enter into the life of another person to accurately perceive their current feelings and meaning. There are many situations in palliative care when patients know that health professionals can not solve their problems, but having the opportunity to voice their concerns maintains hope, and to do this empathy is necessary.

Recognition	Evidence verbally/non-verbally of distress.
Acknowledgement	I understand that you are upset.
Permission	It's okay that you are upset.
Understanding	I would like to explore with you what is making you upset.
Empathic acceptance	You are upset because…
Assessment	Severity and effects of upset.
Alteration (if appropriate)	Removal of upset.
	Cognitive challenge.
	Boosting coping strategies.

Figure 5.3 Handling feelings and emotions.

Hope is a coping strategy used by those confronted with an acute or chronic illness. As Bushkin (5) highlighted, hope is extremely important. Several research studies have addressed the concept of hope and its importance in palliative care. Hope is a difficult concept to measure, and to date a qualitative rather than quantitative research approach has been used in the majority of studies. Communication behaviours clearly influence patients' hope. Koopmeiners *et al.* (23) established that taking time to talk, giving information when requested, being friendly, polite, helpful, and honest as well as just being there, demonstrating caring behaviours were the most important influences on patients' maintenance of hope in a palliative care setting.

Cultural issues in communication

In a multi-culture society communication difficulties may arise with patients when they and their families are from ethnic groups where English is not their first language. These communication difficulties are difficult for staff, as they are unable to accurately assess the patient's understanding of what is being said. The patient may appear to confirm his understanding of what is being discussed with an affirmative gesture, such as a nod. However, this may not be a response to the discussions taking place but may be an instinctive reaction to the patient's embarrassment in failing to comprehend the details of the conversation.

It is thus desirable that every health care organization has easy access to a panel of competent interpreters from whom support is readily available. They often can with close guidance and support, enter into a dialogue with the patient, assess the patient's level of understanding of the present situation, and address his concerns and anxieties.

Observation of the body language and extent of dialogue between the interpreter and the patient is crucial as this can be a reasonable indicator that the interpretations given are those from the patient and not merely perceptions of the interpreter.

An effective interpretation of the situation is fundamental in enabling the patient and family to become fully cognizant of the patient's deterioration and treatment management. This also provides an opportunity for them to ask questions and express their anxieties, concerns, and fears.

In the case where an uncommon language is encountered, and ready access to an interpreter is not available, contact can be made with the appropriate Embassy or High Commission who may be able to advise on appropriate action or supply a suitable contact. This may be time-consuming and the patient may have to wait for some time before a suitable interpreter is located. Therefore other means of communication, such as basic sign language may be adopted to help elicit crucial information to alleviate the patient's and family's anxieties and reassure them that their situation is being addressed and managed.

Communicating with the newly bereaved and issues related to bereavement

The care of the deceased and their relatives should be carried out with respect, dignity, and empathy, and in accordance with the local policy.

The nominated relative(s) should be contacted if they were not present at the time of death and ascertain whether and where (Ward or Chapel of Rest) they wish to view the deceased. If relative(s) or next of kin are not contactable by telephone or by the GP, it may be necessary to inform the police.

Grieving often starts before death as relatives start to experience the pain of their grief. Constant support throughout this time is crucial, particularly immediately following death.

However, it is recognized that many professionals find bereavement difficult to discuss as it may remind individuals of their own personal losses or anticipate future losses; a reminder of one's own and others mortality.

Thus, fears and uneasiness about how the individual professional will act and cope in supporting bereaved relatives' immediate grief and reactions, can affect the way they are managed. If these issues have not been addressed then the bereaved may be left feeling abandoned, isolated, and unsupported. Communication at this time with relatives is therefore crucial.

The communication skills of listening, open questions and empathy, together with the technique for handling emotions and feelings, can be usefully used at this difficult time. Further advice on how or how not to help someone suffering a bereavement is shown in Tables 5.5 and 5.6. Communicating with the bereaved allows relatives to look back over the death of their loved one and ask any questions, thereby facilitating their grieving. It also allows professionals to assess relatives for the risk factors that may complicate a bereavement at a later stage (Table 5.7).

Bereavement can be a particularly stressful time for non-English speaking families. They may have difficulty in making their wishes understood. They may not understand the need for a post-mortem, especially if it conflicts with their religious beliefs. They will need to be given explanations clearly and patiently. They may also need practical advice on funeral arrangements and other legal matters.

In anticipation of the expressive mourning of some ethnic minority families, it may be preferable to provide a secluded ward or room for the people concerned. It may be helpful for ward users if a predetermined maximum number of visitors at any one time is decided. Relatives can be gently reminded of the need to consider other patients.

Table 5.5 How to help someone suffering bereavement[a]

Show	Genuine concern and caring.
Availability	Be on hand to listen and help with whatever they need.
Empathize	Say you are sorry for the death and for their pain.
Expression	Allow the bereaved to express as much feeling as possible; share this with them.
Encourage	Patience; don't expect too much of themselves.
Talk	Allow them to talk about their loss as much and as often as possible.
	Discuss the special or endearing qualities of the deceased.
Reassurance	They did all they could.

[a] Adapted and reproduced from Barbara Ward and Associates (1992), *Good grief; exploring feels, loss and death with over 11's and adults.*

Table 5.6 Areas to be avoided when helping the bereaved[a]

Helplessness	Let one's sense of helplessness keep you from reaching out.
Discomfort/embarrassment	Avoiding them because you are uncomfortable. This adds to the pain; compounding an already painful experience.
Placatory remarks	I know how you feel.
Judgement	Say they ought to be feeling better by now (or similar) which implies a judgement about their feelings.
Block discussion	Change the subject when they mention their loss.
Avoidance/fear of remembrance	Avoid mentioning the loss from fear of reminding them of their pain.
Positive/implications of replacement	Finding something positive about their loss; *at least you have your other* . . . Or *at least you can have another* . . .
Guilt/responsibility for death	Saying anything which may suggest the loss was their fault. There will be enough self-recrimination without further help in this area.
Gratitude	Imply that they should be grateful for either the loss, or for another in their life.
Issue instructions	Tell them what they should do or how they should feel.

[a] Adapted and reproduced from Barbara Ward and Associates (1992), *Good grief; exploring feels, loss and death with over 11's and adults*.

Table 5.7 Pre-bereavement factors that may complicate bereavement

Acceptance Feelings	A relatives' difficulty in accepting diagnosis or prognosis. Relative feels isolated. Relative feels low self-esteem.
Age	Young patient or relative; i.e. child or adolescent.
Prior bereavements	Multiple or previous deaths of close ones. Childhood experience of bereavement.
Relationship with patient	Close/dependant. Ambivalent.
Career	Relative is a member of the caring profession or vocation.
Family	Relative has other dependants; children, parents. Tensions within the family unit.
History	Short or long history of illness. History of mental illness, especially depression.

In every case, attempts must be made to respect the wishes of patients and families, as far as the hospital routine will allow.

The General Practitioner (GP) needs to be informed of his patient's death in order to provide the opportunity of further support to the deceased family, as often the GP is best placed in terms of recognizing the support needs and directing these accordingly.

The other issues that need to be discussed with the patient's relatives are their wishes in relation to Last Offices, jewellery, personal clothing, and any spiritual, religious, or cultural needs, and in some instances it may be necessary to consider possible adjustments in the organization's procedure that will make preparations easier for relatives.

Relatives may also need to be informed about the procedures for collecting the death certificate, registering the death, contacting funeral directors.

The organization's policy must be followed regarding the patient's jewellery, valuables, and belongings. Where appropriate, professionals must check with relatives whether they wish a patient's wedding ring, for example, to be removed.

Any jewellery removed from the patient should be done so in the presence of another professional and recorded along with other valuables on the appropriate documentation and stored according to local policy.

Any family member who removes a patient's belongings must provide a signature for authorization. Any jewellery remaining on the patient should also be recorded on the appropriate form.

The doctor who looked after the deceased will complete a Death Certificate and collection of this must be agreed. Dependent upon circumstances, this may be issued immediately after the death or at a later agreed time. If there is to be a cremation, two certificates, each signed by a different doctor, are required. In the case of a post-mortem, relevant contact numbers and instructions must be given for future advice. In general, a death has to be registered within five days at the Registry of Births, Deaths, and Marriages office in the area where the deceased died.

The bereaved at this difficult time may not be able to take in the necessary information. Therefore they should be provided with appropriate written information on what to do after a death; this should include contact numbers, various help agencies, advice and support on coping with bereavement, and where they may turn to for help.

In summary this chapter has outlined communication issues that commonly arise along the Care Pathway and the benefits of good communication have been highlighted. Unfortunately patients remain dissatisfied with the communication received. However, some programmes of communication skills for health professionals do now appear to be effective in improving communication skills and maintaining levels of skills in the clinical area. The basic skills for good communication have been described and possible techniques for handling the difficult situations have been explored. One of the ways in which health professionals can help themselves to improve their communication skills is to raise their self-awareness of their communication skills by recording an interaction with a patient and listening to themselves. It may be painful to do, but it has to be the responsibility of all working in palliative care as this will go a long way in ensuring that patients are receiving the best care possible, which is the ultimate aim of the LCP.

References

1. King, I. M. (1971). *Towards a theory of nursing*. John Wiley and Sons, Inc., New York.
2. Simpson, M., Buckman, R., Stewart, M., Maguire, P., Lipkin, M., Novack, D., *et al.* (1991). Doctor-patient communication: The Toronto consensus statement. *Br. Med. J.*, 303, 1385–7.
3. Wilkinson, S. M. (1991). Factors which influence how nurses communicate with cancer patients. *J. Adv. Nurs.*, 16, 677–88.
4. Wilson-Barnett, J. (1996). Research directories in palliative care nursing. *Int. J. Palliat. Nurs.*, 2(1), 5–6.
5. Bushkin, E. (1995). Signposts of survivorship. *Oncol. Nurs. Forum*, 22(3), 537–43.
6. Macleod, R. (1991). *Patients with advanced breast cancer: the nature and disclosure of their concerns*. Unpublished MSc Thesis. University of Manchester.
7. Audit Commission. (1993). *What seems to be the matter: communication between hospital and patients*. Audit Commission, National Health Service report no 12.
8. Webb, B. (1995). A study of complaints by patients of different age groups in an NHS trust. *Nurs. Stand.*, 9(42), 34–7.
9. National Cancer Alliance. (1996). *Patient-centred cancer services: What patients say*. National Cancer Alliance, Oxford.
10. Department of Health. (2000). *The NHS cancer plan*. Department of Health, London.
11. Reid, W. (1995). Health Ombudsman Report.
12. Fallowfield, L., Saul, J., and Gilligan, B. (2001). Teaching senior nurses how to teach communication skills in oncology. *Cancer Nurs.*, 24(3), 185–91.
13. Fallowfield, L., Jenkins, V., Farewell, V., Saul, J., Duffy, A., and Eves, R. (2002). Efficacy of a Cancer Research UK communication skills training model for oncologists: a randomised controlled trial. *Lancet*, 359(9307), 650.
14. Wilkinson, S. M., Bailey, K., Aldridge, J., and Roberts, A. (1999). A longitudinal evaluation of a communication skills programme. *Palliat. Med.*, 13, 341–8.
15. Wilkinson, S. M., Roberts, A., and Gambles, M. (2002). The essence of cancer care: the impact of training on nurses' ability to communicate effectively. *J. Adv. Nurs.*, 40(6), 731–8.
16. Wilkinson, S. M., Leliopoulou, C., Gambles, M., and Roberts, A. (2002). Can intensive 3-day programmes improve nurses' communication skills in cancer care? *PsychoOncology*, in press.
17. Hinton, J. (1980). Whom do dying patients tell? *Br. Med. J.*, 281, 1328–30.
18. Quint, J. C. (1967). *The nurse and the dying patient*. Macmillan, New York.
19. Kurtz, S., Silverman, J., and Draper, J. (1998). *Teaching and learning communication skills in medicine*. Radcliffe Medical Press, Oxford.
20. Thompson, D. (1990). Too busy for assessment? *Nurs. J.*, 4(21), 35.
21. Gagan, J. M. (1983). Methodological notes on empathy. *Adv. Nurs. Sci.*, 5(2), 65–72.
22. Kalisch, B. (1973). What is empathy? *Am. J. Nurs.*, 73(9), 1548–52.
23. Koopmeiners, L., Post-White, J., Gutknecht, S., Ceronsky, C., Nickelson, K., Drew, D., *et al.* (1997). How healthcare professionals contribute to hope in patients with cancer. *Oncol. Nurs. Forum*, 24(9), 1507–13.

Chapter 6

Spiritual/religious issues in care of the dying

Peter Speck

How can the Liverpool Care Pathway for the Dying Patient (LCP) influence religious and/or spiritual care?

The essential components of the LCP are: the provision of a means for evaluating outcomes of care, provision of an agreed plan of care to which several professionals may contribute, and the use of current research to establish good practice thereby ensuring that patients receive quality care, especially towards the end of their life. The LCP will provide an effective means of ensuring that this aspect of care for terminally ill patients is effectively taken into account and the appropriate spiritual needs met before and following the death.

Is there a research base for spiritual care in palliative care?

There has been a considerable amount of research in the USA, which has established links between religious affiliation and practice and health outcomes, sense of well-being, mental health, and coping ability. These studies have been undertaken in a culture where the overt practice of religious belief is more prevalent than in the UK. However, studies in the UK into the wider concept of belief indicate that for 69–71% of patients admitted into acute health care, a belief system is important to them and is more predictive of outcome from the illness than the more commonly used psychological measures (1). Studies currently underway indicate that while some people may have moved away from established 'organized' religion they still have an underlying spirituality which is of importance—especially in the course of life crises (2). These studies are in an ageing population, many of whom are aware that their life is entering its final phase.

Why a special focus on spiritual care?

The 'Patient's Charter' in the UK, supported by various NHS guidance letters, and the various codes of good practice for professional groups (such as the UKCC Code for

Nursing) indicate some recognition that this aspect of care is integral to treating patients as people. Spiritual care is widely recognized to be an essential component of specialist palliative care, provided by a multidisciplinary team, as defined by the National Council for Hospice and Specialist Palliative Care Services (3). The integration of the various components of a **holistic** approach includes the psychological and the spiritual (4).

The assessment and provision of these needs may still be somewhat perplexing to health care staff and lead, perhaps, to lip service being paid to this aspect of care, with only the most overt of religious need being addressed. Some of the tools that have been developed so far have either been too lengthy to use, or too tightly within a religious framework in spite of being called a spiritual assessment tool. An integrated care pathway needs to address wider issues than religious affiliation and practice.

What is spiritual care?

'Spiritual' may be described as relating to the vital life essence of an individual. We may not always be consciously aware of its presence or perceive it as an area of need. However, it can assume considerable importance when our physical existence is threatened by disease and death. The outward expression of this vital force or existential dimension will be shaped and influenced by life experience, culture, and other personal factors. It integrates the various aspects of the person and is seen in the quality of relationships. Spirituality will, therefore, be unique for each individual. It may be understood as more than simply a search for meaning, but a search for *existential* meaning within the particular experience or life event, usually with reference to a power other than the self. There may be a developing sense of 'other-ness'. The *existential* dimension is often expressed in terms of questions such as 'Who am I?', 'Does my life have any meaning and purpose?', and 'Has this illness the power to destroy me?' We may not, however, wish to use the term 'God' to describe the power, but may talk about natural or cosmic forces, a sense of the 'other', a power in the universe, etc., which has the ability to enable us to **transcend** the 'here and now' and sustain hope. We may not always choose to express this spirituality through a religious framework.

> Spiritual:
>
> A search for *existential* meaning within a life experience, usually with reference to a power other than the self, not necessarily called 'God', which enables transcendence and hope.

In essence we are talking about ways in which people in times of crisis or other formative moments in their life may become aware of a desire to understand or (existentially) make sense of what they are experiencing.

What is religious care?

A **religion** may be understood as a system of faith and worship which expresses an underlying spirituality.

This faith is frequently interpreted in terms of particular rules, regulations, customs, and practices, as well as the belief content of the named religion. There is a clear acknowledgement of a power other than self, described as 'God' or 'enlightenment'. In some religious understandings this power is seen as an external controlling influence. In others the control is more from within the believer guiding and shaping behaviour. There is a long history of inter-relatedness between religion, healing, and medicine. When talking about religion one would not usually separate religion from spirituality, but neither should one use these terms interchangeably or assume that people who deny any religious affiliation have no spiritual needs. Some people will, therefore, have very clear religious views and needs arising out of their faith perspective. Others will not wish any religious ministry but may value appropriate companionship while exploring their spiritual questioning and needs.

Religious:

A particular system of faith and worship expressive of an underlying spirituality and interpretive of what the named religion understands of 'God' or ultimate reality.

What about people who claim to be neither religious nor spiritual?

For some people the search for existential meaning will take a **philosophical** pathway and exclude any reference to a power other than themselves (e.g. existentialism/ humanism/atheism). The individual, as a product of the individual's own personality and influence, will interpret and influence life events. Atheism, which is the denial of the existence of God, should be distinguished from agnosticism, which allows for a degree of uncertainty as to whether or not a deity exists. Some philosophical people will also claim to be spiritual and to have an appreciation of aesthetic experiences, but would not wish to embrace any notion of an external power that might be influential.

Philosophical:

Where the search for existential meaning excludes any reference to a power other than from the self. Life events and the destiny of the individual being seen as manifestations of the individual's own personality as expressed individually and corporately.

A wider understanding of the word **spiritual, as relating to the search for existential meaning within any given life experience, with the power to transcend that experi-ence,** allows us to consider spiritual needs and issues in the absence of any clear practice of a religion or faith. But this does not mean that they are to be seen as totally separated from each other (5) or that spirituality is a 'wishy-washy' and nebulous concept. At its simplest level it is about affirming and respecting the humanity and 'personhood' of the other person. This becomes important when trying to assess 'spir-itual' need since health care staff may, incorrectly, deduce that those who decline anything religious have no spiritual needs. Frequently, however, the questions that have been asked only relate to religious practice or need and so little attempt has been made to explore the spiritual dimension.

When should we make the assessment?

This care pathway relates to the terminal or dying phase of a person's life and frequently this is not an opportune time to be asking detailed questions, or holding deep philosophical conversations. Some patients are capable and do wish to explore such issues but, as a health care chaplain, I find their ability to sustain such a conversation even when desired is very limited and it has more the feel of 'cramming for finals'.

Ideally, the assessment should be made and reviewed at various points in the illness. At each critical point in the person's life existential questions will arise and will be broached if the patient feels there are people around who will listen, and not leave them feeling 'silly' or morbidly negative.

It is good practice, therefore, for health care staff to have developed a reasonable understanding of where the patient is psychologically, emotionally, and spiritually in terms of their death before the patient enters the terminal phase of their life. This would include the nature of their spiritual/pastoral support needs, their wishes for any (or no) specific religious support or ritual prior to and after death. Clearly needs change and in keeping with good practice in palliative care there should be regular reassessment of all needs over time.

Some people will be very clear and articulate as to their needs while others may become frightened and panicky as they realize their life is drawing to a close.

Sometimes one only meets a patient towards the very end of their life. There may be little opportunity to undertake a detailed assessment of any spiritual needs. If the patient expresses a wish to receive support or help in overcoming any fears or anxieties regarding their future, in terms of the illness or dying, it is important to respond appropriately. This might entail a more formal religious response of prayer, ritual (sacramental or otherwise), offering reassurance, or enabling the individual to express sorrow or sadness for past hurts or misdemeanours. It might also include sitting quietly with the person as they die and, if the carer has a spiritual belief, praying for the dying person and family within one's own heart and mind. Just as there should be regular reassessment of symptoms so there should be ongoing assessment of spiritual need even if the time to death is very short. Any assessment of terminal agitation or pain should include consideration of other factors which could be exacerbating the pain in keeping with the model of 'total pain' (6). It may be too late for the individual to sort out all of the 'unfinished' business in their life. However, they can still benefit from experiencing affirming, accepting care from others whatever their belief system may be.

How can we assess this aspect of people's lives?

Much assessment to date has been of overt religious need with questions about religious affiliation and practice trailing off into silence or confusion if the answers are negative. Clearly there has to be a proper assessment of religious need but there also should be a way of reaching an understanding of what would be helpful for those who are not religious. This should not be an interrogation but more a conversation with a focus that allows key themes to be explored.

Suggested themes (using one's own phraseology) might be:

(a) In the course of your life, with all its ups and downs, have you developed ways of making sense of the things that have happened to you?

(b) When life has been difficult what has helped you cope?

The answer to these questions may highlight the importance of the patient's family, philosophy of life ("I live one day at a time"), or their belief system (religious or spiritual or philosophical), as well as something of their current mental state. Hence it is not pushing people down a narrow religious pathway.

(c) Would you like to talk to someone about the effect your illness is having on you or your family?

Again this does not have to be a religious/faith leader, but when appropriate such a person should be introduced sensitively to patient and family to avoid the stereotypical image of the prelude to death.

*If the conversation indicates that 'belief' is important then staff should enquire what form that belief takes and whether or not it is religious. (N.B. Church of England is a denomination of the religion Christianity and not the religion as so often recorded. In our multi-cultural society we should perhaps now be talking of **Faith Group** and **Faith Leaders** and the **sect/denomination** of that faith group.)*

Strict adherents of a particular faith group may well wish to have opportunity, either privately or with others, to continue to practice that faith. They may also, with their family, have both cultural and faith needs prior to and following their death. The wishes of the family and of the patient may be different and care is needed not to impose onto the patient the family's need. Thus the lapsed Catholic or a Jewish patient has the priest or rabbi 'sent in' by the family, even though he/she does not wish to see the faith leader, and much distress may result.

Each faith tradition has its own rituals and religious practices that can support individuals and enable them to retain and/or strengthen their sense of connectedness with a 'higher power' or God. These religious needs may range from reading passages from the scripture or sacred writings of their faith, to the performance of specific religious rituals such as anointing with oil.

Some religious needs

Prayer and reading of sacred writings

Privately or corporately—prayer time/meditation may require privacy.
Availability of primary texts of the faith tradition.
Commentary and instructive books concerning the faith.

Religious rituals

Initiation rites	e.g. Christian baptism/circumcision.
Holy Communion	Specifically Christian.
Ministry of healing	Laying on of hands, anointing with oil.
Acts of reconciliation and forgiveness.	
Marriage	Either religious ceremony or blessing after civil ceremony.
Corporate acts of worship	Regular, especially on the 'holy' day. At the time of festivals. Funeral/memorial services.
Rites of passage around the time of death.	

What about the needs of different religious/faith groups

It is important that palliative care workers are aware of the importance of a multi-faith approach. They need to consult with the individual to avoid offering care in a stereo-typical way. In reading this section staff must beware the temptation to stereotype (7). Not all adherents of a faith group are equally strict and guidelines are *no substitute* for asking and exploring need with the patient or family. In all cases the family may wish to assist in the performance of Last Offices and may, therefore, appreciate the oppor-tunity to do so.

Anglican and Free Church patients

1. Assurance of spiritual security is vitally important to Christians facing death. A practicing Anglican or Free Church patient will derive spiritual support and com-fort from the presence of a chaplain as death approaches. The chaplain can offer the patient Holy Communion and appropriate prayers, or may simply sit with the patient and relatives to provide spiritual support and comfort.

2. Anglicans have no religious objections to post-mortems and will decide for them-selves in relation to post-mortems not required by law.

3. There are no religious preferences for burial or cremation, it is a matter of indi-vidual choice. However, respect for the body of the deceased is expected from all involved with any procedures following death.

4. It is very important in cases where unbaptized children are seriously ill or near to death that the parents are offered an opportunity to request Baptism for their child. The priest should always be contacted in such cases although a lay person may baptize with water in the name of the Trinity, in the absence of a priest. This applies to all Christians, but some Free Church members who do not sanction infant baptism may wish their child to be named and blessed instead.

Atheists or 'none'

1. If a patient puts 'none' against religion when coming into a health care setting it does not always mean that they have no religious faith. Sometimes it means that they do not wish to be contacted by a chaplain, or asked to make any religious commitment.

2. By creating a sensitive environment in which dying patients can express their feel-ings and fears, staff can fulfil an important pastoral role for patients of no stated religion.

3. However, it is important to understand that a chaplain's ministry has many dimen-sions, one essential element being to build a relationship of trust, understanding, and respect. This must take account of the patient's individual expectations, beliefs, and cultural patterns of behaviour, particularly in times of sickness and death, and make no attempt to impose particular religious views.

4. A sharing of this element of a chaplain's ministry and a gentle introduction of a visiting chaplain, if seen to be appropriate, may do much to comfort the dying patient and bereaved family.

Bahai

1. The Bahai faith is an independent world religion with its own laws and ordinances. Bahais have a great respect for physicians and will wish to consult the best possible medical advice when they are ill.

2. Members are required to say an obligatory prayer each day and read from the scriptures of faith each morning and evening. This practice may continue when a Bahai is dying and should be respected, as should the family or friends' desire to pray with the dying person.

3. Bahais have a great respect for life, believing that their soul progresses after death.

4. There are no ritual procedures for the last offices and unless directed otherwise the usual procedure for the last offices can be carried out. Some families, especially those from an Iranian background, may wish to be present at the washing of the body. This should be respected where possible.

5. There is no objection in the Bahai faith to post-mortem. Bahais are taught to respect the body after death. There is also nothing in their teachings against organ donation.

6. Bahai law forbids cremation, and states that the body should be buried at a site within one hour's journey from the place of death. Bahais are encouraged to include a clause in their will stating their preference for burial.

Buddhist

There are several branches of Buddhism. It is advisable to ask the patient or the family about the nature of any observances to be made.

1. Buddhism stresses the need for the mind to be 'in touch' with the present moment. Buddhists may be distressed if offered drugs that impair consciousness, since great importance is often placed on the conscious state of mind at the time of death. Such medication may be refused.

2. A Buddhist patient may wish to practice 'private meditation' as death approaches. This should be respected where possible.

3. The family will advise on any procedures to be followed, in particular, if a Buddhist monk or sister should be contacted.

4. Where there are no known relatives or at the patient's request, contact can be made with a member of the Buddhist community. Names and telephone numbers should be available on each ward, and also at the back of this booklet.

5. There are no ritual procedures for the last offices. Unless directed otherwise by the family, the usual procedure for the last offices can be carried out.

6. There is normally no objection to post-mortems.

7. By preference, it is usual for Buddhists to be cremated.

The Chinese community

Please discuss the needs of the patient and the family with the individuals concerned.

China has been a communist country for 40 years now and the government has controlled and discouraged any following of religion. However, within China there are practicing Buddhists, Christians, Muslims, and many other faiths. For over two thousand years the teachings of Confucius have guided and shaped the Chinese government and the way that Chinese families have lived. The worship of ancestors became a very important part of Chinese life and it was felt that if respect was shown to elders and ancestors they would receive their blessings. Many Chinese people combine teachings, gods, and beliefs from the three main religions of ancient China: Confucianism, Taoism, and Buddhism. Because of the wide variety of practice and belief it is important to discuss needs with the patient and family.

The Christian faith

The Christian faith is expressed through various denominations that have developed from differences of nationality, historical tradition, temperament, and belief. Individual expectations often vary, not only between the different denominations, but also within them. There are three main Christian denominational groupings in this country with at least one chaplain assigned to each grouping in most health care settings (Church of England/Anglican, Roman Catholic, and Free Church). The common ground between Christian denominations is considerable and enables health care chaplains to work as a team, while recognizing that people's needs may vary according to their Christian tradition.

Special notice should be taken of two of the main sacraments of the Christian Church, Holy Communion and Baptism. Both of these sacraments are available to the patients through a Chaplaincy or Spiritual Care Team. The need to be spiritually prepared for death can be of great importance, often unspoken, to those who may no longer attend formal worship in church.

The chaplain's ministry also extends to caring for the patient's relatives, particularly in times of obvious distress or sudden death, when the presence of the chaplain can bring comfort and support to the grieving family.

Free Church patients

Broadly speaking, the Free Church chaplains are responsible for caring for the spiritual needs of those Christians who are not Roman Catholic or Church of England and their ministry covers members of a wide range of denominations. (A full list can be obtained from Churches Together in England, Tavistock Square, London, UK.) It should be recognized that a patient may also be supported by their own parish priest or Free Church minister who should always be contacted at the patient's/family's request.

Hindu

Hindu beliefs and practices vary considerably. Where at all possible it is advisable to ask the patient or the family about the nature of the particular observances to be carried out.

Most Hindus require time for meditation and prayer, and this will be most evident in terminal illness, when small idols or pictures of gods may be kept under the pillow, or by the bed, as may praying beads and flowers or charms. Recognition should be given to the support, comfort, and help which Hindus derive from these traditions.

Hindu priests very often wish to perform the last rites, but in their absence it would give comfort to the Hindu patient to have some verses from the Bhagavad Gita read to them, if they so desire.

A Hindu priest may be contacted via the family themselves.

1. After the death of the patient, surgical attachments must be removed. Care must be taken *not to remove any threads* which have been put around the neck or wrist by the priest.

2. The body is then left for the family's arrival as they may wish to perform the last offices. It is permissible for the nursing staff to straighten the limbs, close the eyes, and support the jaw if the family have not arrived.

3. As there is usually no restriction on non-Hindus handling the body, and no ritual washing of the body, it is permissible for nursing staff, in consultation with the family to perform the last offices.

4. In circumstances where the family wish to perform the last offices, staff should respect this practice and sensitively offer the family assistance.

5. The body should then be wrapped in a plain *white* sheet and placed in the mortuary. It is acceptable, once the death certificate has been provided, for the relatives to take the deceased home.

6. It is Hindu practice that grief is expressed openly with physical gestures, hands being held and people embracing, much physical comfort being derived from this practice. Staff should provide a quiet place, away from other patients, where the relatives can grieve in this way for an acceptable period of time.

7. Although there are no rules about post-mortems, relatives will often consider them extremely objectionable and disrespectful to the dead. This issue should be handled with great sensitivity when advising Hindu relatives of the need for a post-mortem, e.g. by order of the coroner.

8. It is normal for Hindus to be cremated after death and for the eldest male child to be responsible for the cremation arrangements. Children under five years of age, however, are always buried, never cremated. Staff should be aware of this practice to avoid causing offence or distress to the family.

Jehovah's Witness

1. Jehovah's Witnesses have a high regard for the medical profession and are appreciative of the care and dedication shown to them by health care staff. They are quite willing to accept medical treatment with the *exception* of *blood transfusions* or *blood derivatives*. This stand is based on the command given in the Bible to abstain from taking blood into the body as the life of the donor is within the blood (Leviticus 17: 14 and Acts 15: 20–29). Recent statements indicate that the receipt of blood/blood products in a serious life-threatening event may not always lead to automatic expulsion from the Kingdom Hall. However, this should still be treated with sensitivity.

2. The seriously ill or dying Jehovah's Witness has no morbid fear of death; it is looked upon as a sleep-like condition from which there will eventually be a resurrection as specifically stated in God's word (John 11: 25).

3. The situation may arise where the patient is the only Jehovah's Witness in a family. Care must be taken to handle this situation with the family sensitively if the patient's Presiding Overseer has, *at the patient's request,* been informed.

4. Jehovah's Witnesses do not have any 'last rites' service or similar ministry. It is therefore acceptable for last offices procedure to be followed.

5. There is no particular preference for cremation or burial, it is entirely a matter of individual choice. Jehovah's Witnesses do not usually object to post-mortems.

6. In certain cases, Jehovah's Witnesses nearing death may indicate the wish to donate organs for transplantation. Before taking such a decision, Jehovah's Witnesses would wish for a quiet place to prayerfully consider the matter before making a personal conscientious decision. Staff should be considerate of this and provide a quiet place for them to do this.

Jewish

Jewish beliefs and rites vary considerably with the branch of Judaism to which the person belongs and the degree of Orthodoxy. The wishes of the family should be sought regarding any particular observances to be made.

1. If a Jewish patient is dying, the next of kin should be informed and if it is the wish of the patient and/or relatives contact should be made with the patient's own Rabbi or Synagogue. Similarly, upon the death of a Jewish patient this procedure should be followed. The Rabbi will decide the appropriate form of response.

2. Traditionally the body of the deceased should remain as it was when the death occurred. The body should remain untouched for 30 minutes, during which time surgical attachments should remain in place.

3. Once this period of time has elapsed, if the relatives have not arrived, or it has not been possible to obtain the services of a Jewish chaplain, it is permissible for the nursing staff (*wearing disposable gloves*) to carry out the following procedure.

   (a) The clothes should not be removed.

   (b) The eyes and mouth should be closed. The mouth should be held in a closed position by placing a pillow under the chin.

   (c) The fingers of each hand should be straightened and the hands and arms should be placed parallel to the body. Similarly, the legs and feet should be straightened.

   (d) Any tubes or artificial limbs should be removed and any incisions plugged so as to prevent or stem a flow of blood or body fluids.

   (e) Any *excess* dirt should be wiped away and washed off, but the body should not otherwise be washed.

   (f) The body *still fully clothed* should be wrapped in the bottom sheet. To enable the mortuary technician to respect Jewish tradition, it would be helpful if the body of the deceased could be labelled 'Jewish'. *No* attempt must be made to write on the body as this would cause distress to the relatives.

5. Jewish law requires the body to remain totally intact after death and regards the carrying out of a post-mortem as a desecration of the body. Care should therefore be taken to ensure that the relatives of Jewish patients are not asked to consent to a post-mortem unless required by law, as this is likely to cause offence and distress.

6. Occasionally, a request may be made by members of the family or Jewish community to remain with the deceased either at the bedside or after the body has been removed to the mortuary (a professional 'watcher' may be used). This request is in keeping with Jewish tradition and should be treated with respect.

7. Jewish law insists on the funeral taking place as soon as possible after death, usually within 24 hours. It is therefore important that a death certificate is made available at the earliest possible opportunity, enabling arrangements to commence.

8. Deaths usually have to be registered in the Borough in which they occur. No provision is made by the Registrar within many areas for the registering of deaths on Saturdays, Sundays, and Bank Holidays.

9. While cremation may be more acceptable to some Reformed Jews it is better not to make a reference to cremation unless a relative raises the issue. Burial in a Jewish cemetery is the only option for Orthodox Jews.

10. All still-born babies should be buried and in the event of a miscarriage, the parents should be consulted about the disposal of the fetus to enable them to consult their Rabbi for guidance.

11. In the event of a pregnant woman dying without there being any possibility of safely delivering the child, the mother and child should be buried together without a Caesarian section being performed.

12. It can be a source of considerable comfort to a Jew to know that the staff can say a prayer with them if no immediate family is available.

Mormon

Properly know as 'The Church of Jesus Christ of Latter-Day Saints'.

1. Mormons who have undergone a special Temple Ceremony wear a sacred undergarment. This intensely private item is normally to be worn at all times. It may be removed for laundering or surgical operations but at all times must be considered as *private* and treated with respect.

2. There are no religious objections to blood transfusion.

Diet

Mormons are very health conscious. They are not normally vegetarians, but will only eat meat very sparingly, avoiding products that contain quantities of blood.

They are concerned about stimulants, therefore do not drink tea or coffee. The availability of milk and fruit juices will be appreciated. Alcohol and tobacco are forbidden.

Care for the dying

1. There are no ritual acts for the dying.

2. Contact with other members of the Mormon temple is important.

3. 'Home teachers' will visit and support members.

4. At death, if the sacred garment is worn it must be replaced on the body once last offices are completed.

5. Burial is preferred.

6. A Bishop from the local Mormon Church will be available to give blessings and minister to the sick. The Bishop will offer solace and help with funeral arrangements.

7. Mormons have no religious objections to post-mortem examination or organ donation.

Muslim

It is not always necessary to call an Imam when a Muslim is dying as the family will traditionally stay with the patient to pray. However, if the family is not present, and/or if the patient requests it, contact may be made with an Imam at the local mosque. Muslim beliefs and practices may vary considerably. Where possible it is advisable to ask the family the nature of any observances to be made.

1. Following the death of a Muslim, the body should remain untouched for 30 minutes; surgical attachments, etc. should remain in place.

2. There is usually no objection to non-Muslims handling the body, provided they *wear disposable gloves*. The family may like to perform the last offices themselves and should be consulted in this matter where possible.

3. With the family's approval it is permissible for nursing staff to carry out the following procedure:

   (a) Close the eyes and the mouth. A pillow should be placed under the chin to keep the mouth closed.

   (b) The fingers of each hand should be straightened and the hands and arms should be placed parallel to the body. Similarly, the legs and feet should be straightened.

   (c) Any tubes or artificial limbs should be removed and any incisions plugged so as to prevent a stem or a flow of blood or body fluids.

   (d) Any *excess dirt* should be *wiped* off.

   (e) The head should be turned towards the right shoulder, which will enable the body to be buried facing Mecca.

   (f) The body should be wrapped, *unwashed* and still clothed, in a plain white sheet and placed in the mortuary. It is helpful to denote that the patient is a Muslim on the relevant documentation.

4. Muslim tradition necessitates the washing of the body to be carried out by Muslims of the same sex. This will take place either within the mortuary, at the family home, or sometimes at the mosque.

5. Muslim law insists on the carrying out of a funeral as soon as possible after death, usually within 24 hours. It is important, therefore, that a death certificate be available at the earliest possible opportunity to enable these arrangements to be made.

6. Post-mortems are not usually allowed except by order of the coroner. In other circumstances the next of kin may wish to consult the Islamic authorities before making a decision.

7. Grief may be displayed openly. Staff should endeavour to provide a quiet place for the weeping relatives to grieve for an acceptable period of time, away from patient areas.

8. Muslims are always buried, *never* cremated.

Pagan

The title 'Pagan' does not describe a uniform group but is descriptive of a variety of traditions which have their origins in ancient rituals which are claimed to be more in tune with the elemental forces of the universe. There are many forms of paganism in the UK but the importance of a right relationship with elemental forces is integral to the rituals as well as the health and well-being of the devotee, be they a Druid, a White Wicca, or an adherent of another pagan group. Most members will inform staff of any particular needs.

Sikh

1. If a Sikh patient is dying, the family will wish to be informed at the earliest possible opportunity to enable the following traditions to be followed:

   (a) The priest or family will read hymns to the dying Sikh from the Holy Book—the Adi Granth.

   (b) Before death occurs, a Sikh is given holy water by the priest or family, a few drops being placed in the mouth. Holy water is obtainable from the Temple, or some families will have their own supply brought from the Golden Temple of Amritsar in India.

   A sensitive regard for this practice will bring comfort to the Sikh patient and the grieving relatives.

   In the absence of any relatives, contact can be made with the local Sikh community—the President of the local Sikh Temple will be pleased to advise.

2. After the death of the patient, surgical attachments can be removed and if the family have not arrived it is permissible for the nursing staff to straighten the limbs, close the eyes, and support the jaw. If the family is present, their permission should be sought before carrying out this procedure, as they may wish to do this themselves. Staff should respect this practice, and sensitively offer assistance where appropriate.

3. It is normal Sikh practice for the family to wash and dress the body, such practice usually being carried out at home. However, some Sikh families may wish to carry out this procedure in the place where the person has died. Staff should respect this, and sensitively offer assistance where appropriate.

4. If the family do not wish to carry out the last offices it is permissible for the nursing staff, in consultation with the family, to carry out the following procedure:

   (a) *Wipe* away any *excess* dirt. The body should *not* be washed, unless the family indicate otherwise.

   (b) Plug any incisions to prevent or stem the flow of blood or body fluids.

   (c) The turban worn by male Sikhs should be left in place, as should any small combs which may be in the hair.

   (d) The body should then be wrapped *unwashed* (unless the family has indicated otherwise) in a plain white sheet, and removed to the mortuary.

5. Sikhs are normally cremated, and tradition insists that this take place as soon as possible. Families will be appreciative if the death certificate is available at the earliest possible opportunity.

6. It is usual for still-born babies to be buried, the parents undertaking all the funeral rites.

7. The subject of post-mortem should be treated with sensitivity when advising that this may be required by order of the coroner.

Roman Catholic patients

1. Roman Catholic patients will expect a visit from the priest who may bring Holy Communion and administer the Sacrament of the Sick (Anointing) to those patients who request it. The Anointing is for all those who are suffering from a serious illness, disability, or old age.

2. When a Roman Catholic patient is near to death the priest will also, if possible, give them the Last Rites (Viaticum). This consists of the patient receiving Holy Communion for the last time (Viaticum means 'Bread for the journey'). Once a patient has died, the family may wish the priest to lead the Prayers for the Dead as a last mark of respect and as a support to those who grieve. If in doubt, a priest should always be called, because when a patient states his/her religion to be Roman Catholic, this is what they would usually expect.

What of the non-religious spiritual needs?

The assessment of spiritual need often relates to trying to assess the extent to which the sick person feels disconnected from those people or powers that enable the person to retain some sense of existential meaning and purpose in their life under more normal circumstances. The extent to which we are, or wish to be connected, will depend on previous life experience as well as the present situation or our prognosis for the future. The prospect of imminent or untimely death may well trigger off a lot of **existential questions** for people. The answers to these questions may draw on a belief in a power other than self or not and there is much variety in the understanding of the nature of that power for those who do hold such a belief system. The power may be attributed to God, or it may be expressed through nature and natural forces. More usually it is explored and understood in relationship. People who do not profess any form of religious faith may still wish to have opportunity to be quiet, to reflect, to commune with whatever forces or powers they feel are beneficial to them. In the various ways in which palliative care is made available to people there needs to be opportunity to explore the impact of the

Spiritual pain is liked to:

- A sense of hopelessness.
- Focus on suffering rather than pain.
- Feelings of guilt and/or shame.
- Unresolved anger.
- Inability to trust.
- Lack of inner peace.
- Sense of dis-connectedness or fragmentation.

illness and its consequences for both the quality of life and the ultimate quality of the death event. Spiritual well-being may be a valuable resource to support people as they come to terms with terminal illness and try to retain this sense of identity in the face of illness and treatments which may threaten to fragment it.

Failure to identify and sustain this resource may contribute to the experience of spiritual pain or distress. Spiritual pain is often identified in people whose physical/emotional pain fails to respond adequately to recognized approaches to symptom relief. It is often linked to issues relating to a sense of hopelessness or meaninglessness. It may be expressed as suffering (rather than 'pain') indicating that there seems no meaning or purpose to the pain and the experience is all-encompassing rather than localized or specific. Feelings of guilt or shame may be expressed and an inability to trust—other people, oneself, or 'God'. This can lead to dis-connectedness from a previous religious or belief position, or from other people, which can result in greater *dis*-ease or lack of inner peace. While some of these things can be tackled from a psychosocial perspective, when they assume an ultimate or existential significance the intervention needs to be of a spiritual nature.

The setting in which palliative care is delivered will influence the range of available activities and resources. A home care team may have a more limited opportunity than a day care unit or an in-patient hospice unit. Providing specialist palliative care in a busy acute hospital ward may also restrict what it is possible to provide. It is significant that many of the complimentary forms of therapy have a clear focus on the individual person and on trying to assist that individual in their search for what many describe as 'inner peace' and therefore related to spiritual need and development. Thus aromatherapy, head or foot massage, visualization, or art therapy may all enable the person to explore and express aspects of themselves and their experience of illness and treatment in the hope of transcending some of the more difficult aspects. Reminiscence (written and spoken) and guided imagery are important aspects of care which may help with easing spiritual pain in terms of allowing some healing or reconciliation of the person with their past. Most patients wish to engage in activities which they believe address them more clearly as a person, or which nourish the non-material aspects of their life.

It must not be forgotten that there are also many patients who may not wish to be active but who still value having an aesthetically good setting. For such patients, touch, smell, views through a window, and beauty can become especially important. In this situation it is especially important to focus on the art of *being with* rather than always wanting to be active and *do to*.

Who should meet the needs assessed?

In many cases spiritual care will be the specific remit of properly appointed Faith leaders. Currently these will usually be of a Christian tradition but new guidance on the appointment of health care chaplains will enable Trusts and other health care providers to appoint spiritual care givers from non-Christian traditions where the numbers of patients justify this. Where this is not currently the case those appointed to provide spiritual care should establish links with other faith communities and try to obtain the services of people who can confidently offer supportive care and spiritual support to terminally ill people. The Christian concept of pastoral care is not understood in the same way by some faith groups. For example in Judaism and Islam the faith leader (Rabbi or Imam) would primarily be a teacher who would instruct what to read, what to eat or not eat, or what rituals to follow around the time of death. However, the family or other designated community members would visit to support. In the case of Judaism many of these visitors, however, would studiously avoid talking about the imminent death and direct the individual to thoughts of the goodness of God and blessings of this life. Interpreting the approaches of another culture and faith is fraught with difficulty and we need always to remember we speak from an ethnocentric context however well informed we may be. In all cases the patient should be our guide in terms of need and of who should meet them.

In many cases spiritual care will be provided by the very staff who have assessed it since the patient has developed a trusting relationship with that individual or group. The role of the official pastoral care givers may well be to support the staff as they follow through with the patient rather than taking over. Where very specific rituals are required then faith leader and staff could also work together and complement each other's role at such times.

In many faith traditions the family is the key provider of spiritual support and will often initiate prayers, specific rituals, or requests for more informed or authorized ministry. It is always good practice to consult with the family as to what their wishes may be and this should be a clear component of the LCP.

Acknowledgement

I wish to acknowledge the contribution of Sister Ursula Reynolds Director of Pastoral Care at the Marie Curie Centre, Liverpool, for background research into the religious needs of many of the major faith communities within the UK.

References

1. King, M., Speck, P., and Thomas, A. (1999). The effect of spiritual beliefs on outcome from illness. *Soc. Sci. Med.*, **48**, 1291–9.
2. Coleman, P., McKiernan, F., Mills, M., and Speck, P. (2002). Spiritual beliefs and quality of life: the experience of older bereaved spouses. Quality in Ageing—Policy practice and research (3) 1.20–26.
3. NCHS. www.hospice-spc-council.org.uk
4. World Health Organisation. (1990). Technical Report Series, 804. WHO, Geneva.
5. Speck, P. (1988). *Being there*. SPCK, London.
6. Saunders, C. (1967). *The management of terminal illness*. Arnold, London.
7. Speck, P. (2001). Cultural issues. In *Palliative care for non-cancer patients* (ed. J. M. Addington-Hall and I. J. Higginson). Oxford University Press, Oxford.

Chapter 7

The education strategy to implement the Liverpool Care Pathway for the Dying Patient (LCP)

Deborah Murphy

Introduction

This chapter aims to review the development of an education strategy based on the implementation process of the Liverpool Care Pathway (LCP) into the Acute Hospital Sector. Issues related to the initial implementation process and ongoing core curriculum will be examined. An education programme aimed at the multidisciplinary team (MDT) will be outlined which may be extrapolated to other care settings, e.g. the community.

In every ward area across the Acute Hospital Trust the MDT will encounter death or its aftermath. It is particularly difficult to diagnose whether a patient has entered the dying phase in the acute clinical sector. The shift of focus from that of anti-disease to that of symptom control and ongoing support in the last days or weeks of life can be the most challenging time for a ward team and the educational support in this area of care is generally poor. In ward-based teaching nurses report to us that a 'bad' death can have a lasting impact and leave staff feeling powerless to cope with future death-related issues, a 'good' death can transform practice, improve morale, and impact on future ability to care and indeed shape a nurse's career. It is important to realize that most nursing and medical staff are motivated to provide quality care to patients in the last hours or days of life and that there are often specific factors beyond their control that cause the care of dying patients to be less than adequate. These include lack of appropriate education, 'busyness', and an inappropriate ward environment.

The challenge for the Hospital Specialist Palliative Care Team (HSPCT) is how these concerns, attitudes, and behaviours can be altered to benefit patients, their carers, and the professional clinically-based teams. Education is often delivered away from the clinical arena and context of care and thus away from real life experience of caring for the dying patient and his or her family. This may act as a barrier for the translation of theory into practice in the clinical area. A major cultural shift is required if the needs of dying people are to be met and the workforce is to be empowered to take a leading role in this process. Dying patients are an integral part of the population of general hospitals. Their death must not be considered a failure; the only failure is if a person's death is not as restful and dignified as possible.

We believe that our education strategy and implementation of the LCP has transformed clinical practice. Our proactive approach to the change management process has transformed the care of the dying in the acute hospital sector and goes someway to close the theory/practice gap.

Why do you need to develop an education strategy if you have a valid, reliable, generic, evidence-based document?

The LCP provides a framework, or a blueprint, for practice that is user friendly and evidence based, incorporating specific outcome measures and variance analysis. The culture change required to translate this framework into reality is a more complex issue. Education is key to any process of change if the outcome is to be seen as valid and reliable.

An important part of the role of the Hospital Specialist Palliative Care Team (HSPCT) is to provide education programmes. We have set key strategic targets to outline the role and purpose of our educational agenda:

(a) To empower generic and specialist health care workers within the organization to deliver generic palliative care.

(b) To contribute to the organization's education strategy.

(c) To contribute to postgraduate education in palliative care, external to the organization.

(d) To contribute to nursing/medical undergraduate education programmes.

(e) To disseminate and evaluate education programmes in terms of its effect on clinical practice.

(f) To support staff within the organization in educational initiatives.

It is often difficult to evaluate educational initiatives, particularly if there is no measurable improvement in clinical practice. Education provides the basis for informed decision making, but education alone is of limited value if it is not reflected in clinical practice. The culture of an organization will affect the roles that health care workers play in this decision making process. We believe the culture of care needs to be questioned if we are to sustain any lasting change in care provision. This change must therefore impact on our education strategy. If care needs to be co-operative and reciprocal for it to be empowering then our plan for education needs to be a partnership between the generic worker and the HSPCT.

We also believe that accountability and quality of care are essential components of clinical practice but practitioners cannot provide patients with the best quality of care if they do not know what it is. Knowledge helps practitioners to make more accurate decisions, but knowledge combined with experience provides the key to appropriate decision making. Benner (1) suggests that a strong educational basis is essential to deliver safe care. The progression from novice to expert status assumes that experience will be gained over time, but it must have a firm foundation in education. Acquiring advanced skills in one area of nursing practice will teach professionals how to advance their skills in any area of practice. It is our experience that the more that nurses understand about the dying process and the more influence that nurses feel they have over a situation, the greater the personal effort invested in achieving the desired outcome.

Our challenge was to be sensitive to the needs of our workforce in developing an appropriate educational process. Nurses were particularly keen to learn, but highlighted 'time' as an overwhelming issue; lack of time to give best quality care, lack of time to learn about best practice, and lack of time to make time to 'break the cycle'.

It was unrealistic to think that we could undertake a needs assessment, benchmark current practice, and introduce an educational strategy and culture change across the organization all at once. We chose three pilot areas. These were ward areas that had more than three deaths per month and usually welcomed the support of the HSPCT. We worked with the MDT on these wards over an 18 month period to design the LCP and implement it into their clinical areas and evaluate the process and clinical outcomes. The process we implemented is now recommended to all areas considering emulating this project and will be discussed in the next section.

The 10 step education strategy

In order to introduce the LCP into a specific clinical area, we developed a *ten step* education programme (see Figure 7.1). In a generic setting where a specialist team is based, e.g. hospital or community, this process is likely to take at least 6–12 months to implement. In smaller units including hospices the implementation process can be achieved over a shorter time-scale.

Step 1—Establishing the project

Executive and MDT endorsement for the LCP project

Executive support, i.e. senior management support within the organization is essential for the success of implementing the LCP project. A small group of enthusiastic individuals are unlikely to succeed without executive support. The next step is to gain consensus for the project by the MDT team. This can be done on an individual basis but should include a meeting of the whole MDT. At the initial meeting it is important to discuss with the key players the aims of the LCP project:

(a) To empower generic workers.

(b) To improve care of the dying patient.

(c) To demonstrate outcomes of care for dying patients.

An introduction should also be given regarding key aspects of the LCP including:

(a) Layout of the document.

(b) The importance of diagnosing dying.

(c) The three sections of the LCP:

- ◆ Initial assessment and care.
- ◆ Ongoing care.
- ◆ Care after death.

10 STEP EDUCATION PROGRAMME
MONTH 1

STEP 1—Establishing the project
- Executive and MDT endorsement for the LCP Project.
- Pilot site identified for introduction of the LCP, i.e.—a ward area/unit/department or directorate/GP practice.

Step 2—Development of documentation
- MDT meet to discuss LCP and amend prompts according to local need. N.B.—Goals remain the same.
- Supporting documentation written/identified.

Step 3—Retrospective audit of current documentation
- Optional base review (recommended).

MONTH 2–5

Step 4—Induction—education programme
- Implement intensive education programme over a 6 week period to include all members of the MDT.
- Ensure an LCP resource folder is available to the MDT.

Step 5—Implementation—education programme
- Implement the LCP.
- Provide educational support to staff when patients are cared for on the LCP.

Step 6—Reflective practice
- Review the LCP each time it has been completed and discuss the outcomes of care and completion of the LCP with the MDT on an individual patient basis.

Step 7—Evaluation and training needs analysis
- Evaluate and analyse the LCP—feedback aggregate patient data to MDT.
- Identify specific training or resource needs.

Step 8—Maintenance—education programme
- Regular update teaching sessions according to identified training needs.
- Introduce at least two nurses (registered general nurses grade D–G) from the pilot site to the Palliative Care Team Network Nurse Programme.

MONTH 10–12

Step 9—Training the teachers
- The network nurses depending on prior skill and knowledge are trained to take on the ongoing education role in their own area with the support of the HSPCT: For new staff and ongoing support for the ward team.

Step 10—Programme of ongoing feedback from analysis of the LCP
- Establish a framework of analysis to feedback to staff on a regular basis and to inform the clinical governance agenda.

Figure 7.1 10 step education programme—to facilitate the implementation of the LCP project by an advisory specialist palliative care team.

(d) The LCP is multidisciplinary.

(e) The LCP replaces all previous documentation and is the legal document for patient care.

(f) Explanation of variance and variance analysis.

(g) Benefits of the LCP to the clinical governance agenda.

Pilot site identified for introduction of the LCP, e.g. a ward area/unit/department or directorate/GP practice

It is not possible to implement the LCP project across a large health care setting without first establishing successful pilot sites. This is due to the intensity of the education programme required to successfully implement the LCP.

It is imperative to ensure that the team recognizes that the process of implementation will take time and although at the outset an improvement in care provision will be demonstrated, statistically significant evaluation data will not be achieved in the first six months.

Step 2—Development of documentation

MDT meet to discuss the LCP and amend prompts according to local need

N.B. Goals remain the same.
Each specialist area may have specific needs that are not included. As long as the goals remain the same, the prompts and associated guidelines can be altered to support clinical need.

Supporting documentation written/identified

It is important to have the supporting documentation identified in the LCP available:

(a) Symptom control guidelines.

(b) Facilities leaflet.

(c) Bereavement leaflet.

These may already be available locally. Examples are given in Appendix 5 and 6.

Step 3—Retrospective audit of current documentation

Optional base review (recommended)

A base review is a method of examining current practice. It is a measure of the quality of documentation, not necessarily a measure of quality of care. In this climate of outcome-based care and clinical governance initiatives, it is essential to recognize within your own practice that although care may have been of a high standard, if this has not been documented then in essence care cannot be measured and the intervention did not take place.

We recommend a review of 20 sets of patient clinical notes and suggest examination of cancer-related deaths of patients who have been under the care of an organization for more than 48 hours.

Figure 7.2 is an example of a base review proforma. Figure 7.3 is an example of results from a base review.

The base review is a useful educational tool to demonstrate poor recording of patient care. It is often helpful in persuading more sceptical members of the team the value of the implementing the LCP.

INTEGRATED CARE PATHWAY FOR THE DYING PATIENT PROJECT

BASE REVIEW

49789

This is a scannable form - please complete carefully. Do not staple.
Please refer to guidance notes for completing document

Centre Name

CentreType   Patient Identifier   Pat Age

☐ Hospital   ☐ Hospice   ☐ Community   ☐ Nursing Home

Gender (Please circle)   Admit Date   Death Date

M   F

Primary Diagnosis - please refer to data dictionary (please tick only one)

Cancers:

☐ Bone (sarcoma)	☐ Liver	**Non cancers**
☐ Breast	☐ Pancreas	☐ Acute abdomen
☐ Eye	☐ Penis	☐ Arthritis
☐ Meninges	☐ Prostate	☐ MI, CCF
☐ Brain	☐ Testis	☐ Stroke
☐ Anus	☐ Mesothelioma	☐ Alzheimers
☐ Colon	☐ Other connective/soft tissue disorders	☐ Epilepsy
☐ Oesophagus	☐ Bronchus	☐ Motor neurone disease
☐ Rectum	☐ Non small cell lung	☐ MS
☐ Small intestine	☐ Small cell lung	☐ Parkinsons disease
☐ Stomach	☐ Trachea	☐ CNS: other
☐ Adrenal	☐ Malignant melanoma	☐ Hepatobiliary
☐ Carcinoid	☐ Non melanoma	☐ HIV/AIDS
☐ Neuroendocrine	☐ Bladder	☐ Renal
☐ Thyroid	☐ Kidney	☐ Respiratory
☐ ENT	☐ Ureter	☐ Vascular
☐ Female genital organs	☐ Cancer of primary multiple sites	☐ Other non cancer
☐ Leukaemia	☐ Unknown primary	
☐ Lymphoma	☐ Other cancer	
☐ MDS		
☐ Myeloma		
☐ Gall bladder		

> **For "Patient Identifier" please enter a number which uniquely identifies your patient. Please enter it on each page in proforma**

Figure 7.2 Base review proforma.

49789

Patient Identifier

COMFORT MEASURES

1.1 Pats current medication assessed and non essentials discontinued ☐ Yes ☐ No

1.2 If other medication not discontinued was a documented reason given ☐ Yes ☐ No

2 Was as required (PRN) prescribed subcutaneously:	2.1 Analgesic	☐ Yes ☐ No	2.2 Antiemetic	☐ Yes ☐ No
	2.3 Anticholinergic	☐ Yes ☐ No	2.4 Sedative	☐ Yes ☐ No

2.5 If yes were drugs prescribed the ones recommended in your local formulary guidelines ☐ Yes ☐ No

3 Were the following interventions discontinued	3.1 Blood Tests	☐ Yes ☐ No ☐ Not applicable
	3.2 Antibiotics	☐ Yes ☐ No ☐ Not applicable
	3.3 Intravenous fluids	☐ Yes ☐ No ☐ Not applicable

3.4 Were do not resuscitate instructions documented ☐ Yes ☐ No ☐ Not applicable

3.5 Were instructions re do not transfer to hospital documented ☐ Yes ☐ No ☐ Not applicable

3a Were inappropriate nursing interventions discontinued:

3a.1 Routine Turning Regime ☐ Yes ☐ No ☐ Not applicable

3a.2 Taking vital signs ☐ Yes ☐ No ☐ Not applicable

3b Was a syringe driver set up within 4 hours of prescription ☐ Yes ☐ No ☐ Not applicable

PSYCHOLOGICAL/ INSIGHT ISSUES

4 Ability to communicate in English Assessed ☐ Yes ☐ No ☐ Not applicable

5.1 Patient aware of diagnosis? ☐ Yes ☐ No

5.2 If no is there a documented reason ☐ Yes ☐ No ☐ Not applicable

5.3 Patient aware s/he is dying ☐ Yes ☐ No

5.4 Next of kin aware patient is dying ☐ Yes ☐ No

RELIGIOUS NEEDS

6.1 Patients religious needs assessed ☐ Yes ☐ No ☐ Not applicable

6.2 Patients religious needs met ☐ Yes ☐ No ☐ Not applicable

COMMUNICATION WITH FAMILY - OTHERS - PRIMARY HEALTH CARE TEAM

7 Identified how family/others were to be contacted/ informed of patients impending death? ☐ Yes ☐ No ☐ Not applicable

8 Family/others given written information re facilities ☐ Yes ☐ No ☐ Not applicable

9 Patients GP/locum service aware that patient in dying phase ☐ Yes ☐ No

10 Patients plan of care discussed with family/others ☐ Yes ☐ No ☐ Not applicable

Figure 7.2 Continued.

49789

Patient Identifier

| | | | | |

SECTION 2: ONGOING ASSESSMENTS

S2.1 Assessment of pain 4 hourly/each visit   ☐ Yes   ☐ No

S2.2 Was the patient in pain   ☐ Yes   ☐ No

S2.3 Was prn analgesia given   ☐ Yes   ☐ No

S2.4 Assessment of nausea & vomiting 4 hourly/each visit   ☐ Yes   ☐ No

S2.5 Was nausea & vomiting a problem   ☐ Yes   ☐ No

S2.6 Was prn antiemetic given   ☐ Yes   ☐ No

S2.7 Assessment of Agitation 4 hourly/each visit   ☐ Yes   ☐ No

S2.8 Was agitation a problem   ☐ Yes   ☐ No

S2.9 Was prn sedation given   ☐ Yes   ☐ No

S2.10 Assessment of excessive respiratory secretions 4 hourly/ each visit   ☐ Yes   ☐ No

S2.11 Was excessive respiratory secretions a problem   ☐ Yes   ☐ No

S2.12 Was prn anticholinergic given   ☐ Yes   ☐ No

S2.13 Assessment of mouth care 4 hourly/each visit   ☐ Yes   ☐ No

S2.14 Assessment of Micturition problems 4 hourly/each visit   ☐ Yes   ☐ No

S2.15 If pressure relieving aids required were these provided   ☐ Yes   ☐ No

S2.16 Assessment of Bowel Care 12 hourly/each visit   ☐ Yes   ☐ No

CARE AFTER DEATH

S3.1 GP/Locum Service contacted re patients death   ☐ Yes   ☐ No

S3.2 Post mortem discussed   ☐ Yes   ☐ No   ☐ Not applicable

S3.3 Special needs identified /religions / infection needs   ☐ Yes   ☐ No

S3.4 Family/others informed of tasks following death   ☐ Yes   ☐ No

S3.5 Appropriate documentation given to family/others   ☐ Yes   ☐ No

Figure 7.2 Continued.

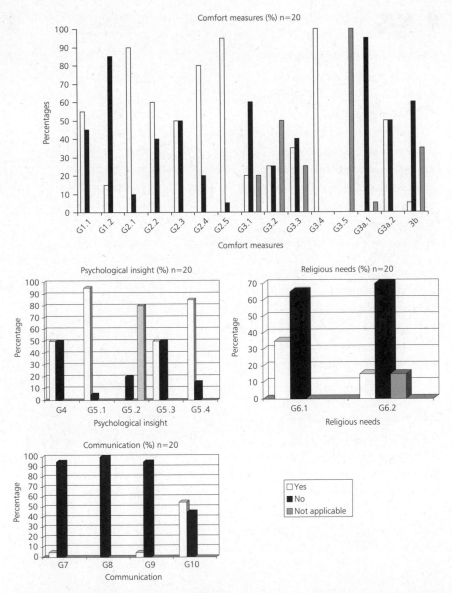

Figure 7.3 Results from a base review related to the goals in the initial assessment and care of the LCP, based on 20 patients case notes.

Of the 10 initial assessment goals four goals were recorded as achieved in over 50% of patients:

Goal 1—Current medication assessed and non-essentials discontinued.

Goal 2—PRN subcutaneous medication written up.

Goal 5—Patient/family recognition of dying.

Goal 10—Plan of care discussed with family/other.

Six goals were recorded as achieved in less than 50% of patients:

Goal 3—Discontinue inappropriate interventions.

Goal 4—Ability to communicate in English assessed which was poorly recorded.

Goal 6—Religious needs identified.

Goal 7—Identified how family is to be informed of patient's impending death.

Goal 8—Family given information on facilities.

Goal 9—GP practice aware of patient's deteriorating condition.

Step 4—Induction—education programme

Implement intensive education programme over a six week period to include all members of the MDT

Each time the LCP is introduced into a clinical area it will take four to six weeks to include all the relevant personnel in the education programme. An outline of the learning outcomes are identified in Figure 7.4. In the acute sector it usually takes at least two to three, 30 minute teaching sessions with associated learning outcomes per week. This can be either one to one or in small groups of staff in order to capture the entire ward team.

Ensure an LCP resource folder is available to the MDT

A resource folder should be available in the pilot area. It should contain relevant evidence-based documentation and guidance to inform users of the LCP. A suitable starting point for constructing a resource folder would be using the reference list from the relevant chapters in this book.

Step 5—Implementation—education programme

Implement the LCP

Once the majority of the team has undertaken the appropriate teaching sessions the LCP can be piloted. Clearly this initial period will require maximum support from the HSPCT. A specialist nurse may need to dedicate up to one-third of his/her available time to achieve this. It is this initial process and the high profile and availability of a member of the HSPCT that is the key to the ongoing success of the project. It would appear that the process of a specialist resource coming to the clinical area and working in tandem with the generic team enhances both knowledge and confidence and supports the transfer of this new knowledge into clinical practice.

Provide educational support to staff when patients are cared for on the LCP

Each time the LCP is utilized the ward contacts the HSPCT and a member of the team visits the ward area irrespective of clinical need. The supportive role of the HSPCT allows for ongoing discussion of individual patients and specific problems and encourages discussion within the ward area of potentially difficult issues. There are occasions where education alone cannot achieve optimum care and confidence to practice must be considered.

Induction—education programme—learning outcomes:
Each health care worker will be able to:

1. Describe the reasons for the introduction of the LCP.
2. Clearly identify criteria for initiating the LCP.
3. Describe the three sections of the LCP.
4. Assess symptoms in dying patients.
5. Interpret the symptom control guidelines.
6. Communicate appropriately with patients and relatives.
7. Assess religious/spiritual needs.
8. Appreciate the need for accurate documentation and variance recording.
9. Demonstrate that once initiated the LCP replaces all other documentation and becomes the single record of care.
10. Access relevant supporting documentation in the ward area.
11. Contact the Hospital Specialist Palliative Care Team (HSPCT) initially each time the LCP is used.
12. Access the palliative care resource folder in the ward area.

Figure 7.4 An outline of the learning outcomes from an education programme.

Step 6—Reflective practice

Review the LCP each time it has been completed and discuss the outcomes of care and completion of the LCP with the MDT on an individual patient basis

After each occasion in the first few months when a LCP is utilized the HSPCT will liaise directly with the ward team to discuss an individual case so that encouragement is given and any problems discussed in real time. This nurturing further encourages the empowerment of the ward team and helps them recognize the value of the change process and their very specific valuable contribution. Increased knowledge and confidence to practice has empowered the MDT to adopt a more questioning approach to care provision.

One very specific example of how a lack of confidence in practice influences patient care was highlighted during a supportive visit to a ward area by a Macmillan Palliative Care Nurse Specialist. One of the ward staff commented how difficult she and her colleagues had found an individual patient. This patient was assessed accordingly and was restless and agitated in the last hours of life. Whilst the staff had assessed the patient status appropriately and were aware of the most appropriate action to be taken, the fear of giving an injection that they knew would resolve the symptoms was overwhelming and the relevant medication was not given.

This fear and lack of confidence was reflected upon with the staff. The fear of the patient dying immediately following an injection was overwhelming. The staff reported that they were concerned that there would be repercussions from relatives and their inability to deal with this discussion was highlighted. The regular support of the HSPCT allows the practitioner to discuss fears or concerns in a non-threatening one-to-one discussion which increases confidence and empowers the individual. It is therefore ultimately this empowerment of the individual that will sustain a change in practice. We do not believe that this reflection on practice and admission of fear and confidence issues would have been raised prior to LCP implementation. It appeared that we had created a supportive environment for reflective practice and altered the previous culture or practice.

It is also important to ensure that if specific areas of research-based practice have been highlighted that the relevant guidelines and articles are available in the resource folder for reference.

Step 7—Evaluation and training needs analysis

Evaluate and analyse the LCP—feedback aggregate patient data to the MDT

Chapter 9 describes the evaluation process and illustrates the type of information that can be fed back to staff. This includes highlighting areas of high achievement and also identifies areas in need of additional training and resources.

Identify specific training or resource needs

For example a goal is set to assess and undertake appropriate mouth care at least every four hours. In fact the ward team did not have the equipment required. The LCP highlighted this issue and lead to use of a problem solving model to enable the network nurses to change the Trust mouth care policy and obtain appropriate mouth swabs available as stock items on all wards.

The LCP also highlighted educational concerns re communication with relatives and carers. Staff were aware of the need to assess insight levels of carers but did not feel competent to undertake this issue. We were able to modify our training programme to support communication skills training.

Step 8—Maintenance—education programme

Regular update teaching sessions according to identified training needs

An ongoing teaching programme is established following discussion with the network nurses and ward team. Key areas will need to be reviewed by the HSPCT as required but every six months a reassessment-needs analysis is undertaken in support of specific requirements.

Introduce at least two nurses (registered general nurses grade D–G) from the pilot site to the Palliative Care Team Network Nurse Programme

Once we had undertaken the pilot project across three ward areas, key members of staff who had become natural leaders of the project management in their own areas expressed a wish to meet with other nurses to share knowledge of this project. These nurses also expressed a desire to learn more about the palliative care approach and to help develop a more robust education programme for learning within the clinical area and asked us if we could facilitate this. The HSPCT had previously attempted to develop a link nurse programme but systems introduced had not been sustainable. It would appear that the implementation process for the LCP had in some way captured the vision and imagination of the generic health care worker.

The programme adopted is known as the Palliative Care Team Network Nurse Programme and it has further transformed our educational initiatives.

It is our experience that by month seven to nine, the team will be more than capable of using this document in the main without the direct support of the HSPCT. If not previously, then at least at month seven the ward area will nominate two members of the ward team to join the network nurse programme. Whilst the majority of members will be nurses as they lead clinical practice development in the clinical areas, all other members of the MDT are welcome.

The role of the network nurse

(a) To have or acquire knowledge and skills in the palliative care approach.

(b) To be willing to share knowledge and skills with other generic workers in the ward environment.

(c) To take a lead role in the support and management of patients with palliative care needs on their ward.

(d) To liaise regularly and be supported by the relevant Macmillan Palliative Care Nurse Specialist.

Step 9—Training the teachers

The network nurse depending on prior skill and knowledge is trained to take on the ongoing education role in their own area with the support of the HSPCT:

◆ For new staff.

◆ Ongoing support for ward team.

The development of a core curriculum in the palliative care approach for the network nurses, or an ongoing education programme to sustain the LCP project and develop the skills of the generic worker in the clinical area, needs to be considered. We designed our programme in line with the needs of the workforce and the needs of the HSPCT in order to reflect our expectations of the generic worker and in line with our referral criteria.

It is the responsibility of every health care professional to provide palliative care and to call in specialist colleagues should the need arise as an integral component of good clinical practice, whatever the illness or its stage. Our key educational role is to facilitate and empower the Network Nurse and the generic worker in the palliative care approach, to support the Network Nurse, to assess, plan, and implement care, and to work together to achieve symptom management. We should also support communication skills, e.g. broaching and exploring the subject of cancer and dying—exploring feelings and answering patients difficult questions.

Core curriculum—network nurse programme

◆ Management of pain.

◆ Management of other symptoms, e.g. nausea.

- Psychological support for the patient and carer.
- Care of the dying/distressed.
- Insight of the patient/carer.
- Complex placement issues.
- To maintain use of the LCP on the ward.

What are the advantages of being a Network Nurse?

1. Empowering the team where you work.
2. Enhancing the skills of you and others.
3. Free place at a National Palliative Care Conference.
4. Potential opportunity for financial support for self-education/study.
5. Network badge/certificate.
6. Opportunity to be part of a wider network in palliative care in the future.

Step 10—Programme of ongoing feedback from analysis of the LCP

Evaluation of ongoing LCP outcome data is collated and disseminated to the network nurse and the ward team on a regular basis. This is essential to maintain the momentum of the project and continue to support the ongoing education programme with robust variance reporting. The ward team may decide to share data across teams or a directorate, which in turn enhances liaison and feeds into the clinical governance agenda (see Chapter 9).

What was the impact on the HSPCT of the LCP educational strategy?

Petty and Cacioppo (2) identified that understanding attitudes is important because it provides insight into what can be expected of others. This is significant because the intention to perform a given behaviour is influenced by personal and social factors. Personal factors include an individual's attitude towards certain behaviour, while social factors include the social pressure to perform that behaviour (3). Other factors to consider are the influences of knowledge, skills, time, opportunity, autonomy, and resources, all of which affect behavioural intent (4).

The HSPCT needed to have some degree of insight into the influences and stressors felt by the ward team and the best ways to influence behaviour. This is not a skill inherent in the development of a HSPCT and the needs of the team must be considered if we are to work in partnership to change behaviour and sustain the process.

The experience of this project has influenced how we work as a HSPCT. We now recognize the importance of educating according to need and at an appropriate and often basic level. If we are to practice at a specialist level then we must empower and educate at the generic level, with specific emphasis on teaching within the clinical area. The power of a specialist resource in the clinical area (irrespective of need) to influence and change practice can not be overstated.

How do you know that your education programme has been successful?

Evaluation of any education initiative is always difficult. Whilst teaching sessions may be enjoyable and learning outcomes set and achieved, a demonstrable change in clinical practice is of paramount importance and is not as easily achieved or measured. We can demonstrate statistically a reduction in basic and inappropriate referrals to the HSPCT so our specialist input has significantly increased. We have rationalized our educational input to include more specific interventions that will continue to change practice.

The ward teams have been empowered to support the HSPCT in ongoing initiatives, taking part in teaching themselves. These nurses report to us that they would not have had the confidence to do this without the LCP programme.

The network nurse programme has been sustained and is a model adopted by other specialties within and without the university hospitals to empower and educate the generic worker. Care of the dying has been transformed across the organization.

This translation of theory into practice has been applied by ward teams to other elements of care. The way we interact with people has a direct consequence on their behaviour, well-being, and self-esteem. We can clearly demonstrate that the supportive and palliative care approach we have instilled into our workforce has impacted on the culture of the organization.

Conclusion

We believe that our project has been successful because we have consulted, co-operated, and collaborated with the generic workforce at every stage. We have achieved our vision to introduce an evidence-based, outcome-led document in the care of patients and their carers in the last days of life. We have demonstrated a process that inspires, motivates, and truly empowers the generic workforce promoting the educational and empowerment role of the HSPCT. This generic clinically-based education programme has enhanced clinical care and communication skills and ensured that the process and outcome is meaningful and sustainable at ward level.

Stevenson and Parsloe (5) state: "Empowerment is about processes which permeate organisations and professional thought, the challenge is to create a culture in which such processes are able to thrive." We believe the LCP education project empowers doctors and nurses to deliver high quality care to dying patients and their relatives.

References

1. **Benner, P.** (ed.) (1984). *Uncovering the knowledge embedded in clinical nursing practice.* Addison Wesley.
2. **Petty, R. and Cacioppo, J.** (ed.) (1996). Introduction to attitude and persuasion. In *Attitudes and persuasion: Classis and contemporary approaches.* Boulder Co, Westview Press.
3. **Ajzen, I. and Madden, T.** (1986). Prediction of goal-directed behaviour: attitudes, intentions and perceived behavioural control. *J. Exp. Soc. Psychol.*, **22**, 453–74.
4. **Nash, R., Edwards, H., and Nebauer, M.** (1993). Effect of attitudes, subjective norms and perceived control on nurses' intention to assess patient's pain. *J. Adv. Nurs.*, **18**(6), 941–7.
5. **Stevenson, O. and Parsloe, P.** (1993). *Community care and empowerment.* Rowntree, York.

Chapter 8

Implementing the Liverpool Care Pathway for the Dying Patient (LCP) in hospital, hospice, community, and nursing home

Alison Foster, Elaine Rosser, Margaret Kendall, and Kim Barrow

In the hospital—Alison Foster

Why implement the LCP in the hospital setting?

The process of developing the LCP involved the time and resources of an energetic and committed team of people. Our vision in developing the LCP across the continuum of health care settings was to identify the needs of dying patients and their families, in the hospital, hospice, nursing home, and community. Initially the LCP was developed to translate the hospice model of best practice into the acute hospital setting. It was hoped that this would transform and improve the quality of care of the dying patient and their family.

Most patients die in an acute hospital setting. The Office of Population Census and Surveys 2000 (1) revealed that of all deaths 67% occur in hospital, 29% in the community, and 4% in a hospice. Since these statistics are unlikely to radically alter in the near future, it is essential to focus on ways in which care of the dying in the acute sector can be improved. The development of Hospital Specialist Palliative Care Teams (HSPCT) and improved medical and nursing undergraduate training have recently improved the care of the dying (2). However, despite the rapid growth and integration of HSPCTs over the last decade, it is unrealistic to expect them to care for all dying patients within their organization. For example, The Royal Liverpool University Hospitals Trust has approximately 2000 deaths per year. The HSPCT is currently involved in the care of 15% of patients dying in the Trust. It is therefore the HSPCTs responsibility to provide education and evidence/research-based guidelines of best practice for the generic multidisciplinary team, to empower them to care for the 85% of dying patients whom the HSPCT are not directly involved with.

What does implementation of the LCP in the hospital involve?

A multidisciplinary working party was formed to consider how best to adopt the culture of care pathways into the specific palliative care needs of patients dying in the acute hospital setting. Members of the working party included: Macmillan Palliative Care Nurse Specialists, a Consultant in Palliative Medicine, a Care Pathways Manager, members of the ward teams, representatives from the pastoral care team and general office, and a pharmacist. Also there was further consultation with hospice, community, and nursing home palliative care specialists. It is important to emphasize the value of seeking executive endorsement and support from within your organization at the early stage of implementation. The working party also discussed and identified the key stages necessary for successful implementation and developed a strategy to meet these needs. The strategy comprised six areas (these have been further developed into the Ten step education strategy described in Chapter 7) which are discussed in more detail below:

◆ Base review.

◆ Supporting documentation.

◆ Education programme.

◆ Pilot study.

◆ Implementation and ongoing support.

◆ Audit and feedback.

Base review

A review of previous and current practice was undertaken to provide a baseline of the current level of knowledge and practice within the trust to enable a comparison to be made post-implementation. The base review involved the retrospective study of a random selection of 20 sets of patients' case notes focusing on the patients' last 48 hours of life. A proforma based on the goals and outcomes specified in the LCP, was developed to record the data collected. The difficulty with the base review was that since documentation was so fragmented, it was challenging to establish what care the patients had actually received during the last days of life. Findings demonstrated areas for concern such as poor and inappropriate symptom control. For example, diamorphine was routinely given for agitation and distress rather than a benzodiazepine. There was also no evidence of anticipatory prescribing and there were examples of inappropriate interventions. For example, intravenous hydration was continued until death in the majority of patients. Poor communication with the primary health care team and little documentation of spiritual and religious support were also noted. However, it is important to mention that the base review also highlighted good practice.

A confidential questionnaire was distributed to all auxiliary, qualified nursing and medical staff to ascertain their knowledge base and give them an opportunity to express how effective they felt they were in caring for dying patients and what they felt could be improved. There was a 70% response rate. The results highlighted the need for education concerning symptom control in the dying patient. However, some ward staff felt what they needed most of all was access to more Macmillan nurses rather than access to relevant education and guidelines of best practice.

Supporting documentation

A number of supporting documents were identified/developed and made available to all ward areas in the form of a resource folder. The documents underpinned the goals identified in the LCP and ranged from local policies and guidelines to national publications.

Specific information to support the patient's family/other was also identified and developed, comprising:

+ Hospital facilities and accommodation leaflet.

+ Bereavement leaflet.

+ What to do after a death—DSS (3).

+ Hospital general office booklet.

Education programme

It was evident from the outset that ward staff would require encouragement, help, and support to ensure effective use of the LCP. However, this alone was not sufficient. The culture and attitude of a workforce suffering from poor morale, continual pressure, and lack of time also needed to be addressed (4) to truly empower the generic worker and bridge the theory/practice gap.

Initially, two key nurses from each ward area were invited to attend a study day, followed by regular meetings. The key nurses' responsibility was to disseminate their knowledge to their colleagues. This strategy was unsuccessful because the information did not filter through to the ward area and the care pathways were only being used when the key nurses were on duty.

As a result a new strategy was implemented. It seemed that it would be more effective to allow all nurses access to a short ward-based teaching session. The reformed education programme included the nomination of two key nurses from each ward to assist with LCP implementation, repeated compulsory 30 minute planned teaching sessions for all nursing staff within a four to six week period. Training sessions were included within the induction programmes of newly appointed and overseas nurses.

The education of junior medical staff was challenging due to inherent difficulties and time constraints. It was decided to give them an opportunity to learn about the LCP in a variety of ways. For example, one-to-one ward-based teaching and teaching during their pre- and post-registration tutorials. Senior medical staff gained information during presentations at multidisciplinary and clinical governance meetings and Grand Round presentations.

It is important to note that a commitment to ongoing education is crucial after the LCP has been implemented to sustain the project. We also identified other related educational requirements as a consequence of our increased profile in the ward areas.

Pilot study

A pilot study was conducted on three medical and wards and three surgical wards. We chose wards that had a high mortality rate, where we felt that the LCP would have greatest impact, and where the HSPCT already had a high profile. The pilot allowed maximum support to be given to wards using the LCP and also thorough evaluation of its implementation.

Permission was sought from the relevant managers and consultants to launch the LCP with a view to obtaining blanket approval and consensus. There was a strong element of interest and support with few objections raised.

Once the pilot study began, regular meetings were held with the multidisciplinary working party and ward staff. As a result the LCP was refined into its present format.

Implementation and ongoing support

Once the educational programme and pilot study were completed, the LCP was ready to be launched. A strategy comprising specified milestones over a 12 month period was developed to provide a supportive structure and framework for ward staff to facilitate smooth implementation of the LCP. This is outlined in the education chapter.

The milestones include working with the nominated key nurses, making daily ward visits to answer queries, and develop ward staff's knowledge and confidence. Feedback of variance analysis and audit to key nurse/ward team is also a key part of the education package. It is useful to monitor the number of deaths occurring on the ward, to enable staff to see how many patients had been put on the LCP, and if a patient had not been put on the pathway to establish why not.

After six months implementation, data analysis should be presented back to the ward team so that the information cycle is complete and staff begin to develop a sense of ownership of the LCP project. It is beneficial to provide staff with a forum in which they can discuss specific anecdotal data and evaluate experience. To undertake a post-implementation review may also be helpful at this stage, to compare results with the initial base review.

Over this period of time it is likely that the wards will develop autonomy using the LCP. Less input is required from the HSPCT. However, it is imperative to formalize a plan with the key nurse/multidisciplinary team to sustain the project.

The team co-ordinating the project may then focus on another area in which to implement the LCP. It is our experience that it would not be possible to launch the LCP across the all wards of the hospital at the same time, as it is likely that there would not be the manpower available to support implementation sufficiently.

Audit and feedback

Audit and variance analysis are vital aspects of the LCP cycle. Pre-implementation, the identification of the audit process and manpower cannot be stressed highly enough. This was one of our biggest challenges. However, we are now fortunate to have designated audit time from within the Trust. Another important practical note is to ensure that systems are in place to trace and obtain the LCPs from the medical notes once they are completed. Not being able to find the LCPs makes audit impossible.

Analysis based on data collected from the pilot ward demonstrated favourable outcomes which, when compared to those achieved in the hospice setting were similar. Significant improvements were evident when the outcomes were compared to the initial base review. This data suggests that the LCP had improved the care of the dying patient in the hospital setting.

What are the specific challenges of implementing the LCP in the hospital?

We encountered many challenges along the way, the majority of which were anticipated but needed careful, sensitive consideration to overcome them.

1. From the perspective of the ward team, the most difficult dilemma for the nurses and clinicians was to know when to use the LCP and diagnose dying. This is particularly difficult when patients have been acutely ill or in a post-operative state, or indeed, for some patients with a non-malignant disease where the disease trajectory may be unpredictable. The ward team should be reassured that the LCP is not one way and if a patient's condition improves the LCP can be discontinued.

2. Occasionally negative attitudes were encountered. For example, the LCP was perceived as 'cookbook medicine that discouraged appropriate clinical judgement from being applied in individual patient's care'. Opinions such as these usually stem from a lack of understanding and experience, highlighting a need for education.

3. Some nursing staff found it difficult to accept that the LCP replaced all other forms of documentation, such as the nursing Kardex, and some were under the misapprehension that they had to complete both.

4. Occasionally staff working within highly specialized areas of health care questioned what the LCP could teach them about improving the care they give to their patients. This is understandable but it is relevant to demonstrate the other benefits of using LCPs, for example the ability to demonstrate quality of care, and meeting clinical governance requirements.

5. The HSPCT had unrealistic expectations of how many deaths we would encompass within the LCP. We have since learned that there can be valid reasons why the LCP is not used, for example in the case of a sudden death, a cardiac arrest, or difficulty in diagnosing dying, or perhaps simply a member of staff being unfamiliar with the tool.

6. The biggest challenge was that we did not realize how costly this project was going to be, in terms of time, manpower, and sustenance. However, after five years working with the project, we are reaping the benefits. More importantly, the patients and their families who die within our Trust are reaping the benefits, together with the staff who care for them.

What are the benefits for the hospital setting?

The benefits of implementing the LCP are numerous, far exceeding our expectations. At ward level, implementation of the LCP improved documentation and communication within the multidisciplinary team, promoting teamwork. It also enhanced communication between health care professionals and patients. By generating outcomes of care, the LCP demonstrated quality of care and provided a mechanism for audit leading to the identification of future research and development questions. It is also a useful tool to demonstrate to purchasers and users of the service the standards achieved regarding care of the dying in line with the NHS cancer plan (5).

The benefits to the ward teams are that the LCP appears to encourage successful teamwork, communication, and care planning. There is less time spent on paperwork, freeing more time to deliver patient care. The LCP provides a framework that enables staff to deal with situations they may have found difficult previously, developing a sense of empowerment, safe in the knowledge that they are delivering high quality evidence-based care. This is enormously valuable not only when caring for a particular patient but in strengthening a sense of purpose, morale, and satisfaction in staff.

Feedback of data informs staff of good practice. This is very important in the acute health care setting when staff often feel undervalued. The number of complaints related to death and dying within the hospital has fallen since implementation of the LCP.

In addition to being a powerful education tool, the LCP has contributed to the development of the palliative care Network Nurse Programme (NNP), which aims to promote an improved and integrated service. It promotes a forum for continual, shared learning to improve care for patients who need a palliative care approach (6).

The impact upon the HSPCT is demonstrated by the reduction in the number of referrals to the team. The referrals are now more complex in nature and utilize more appropriately the expertise of the specialist team. In addition, data analysis identifies research and development questions that will have a direct impact upon patient care, together with demonstrable outcomes of care.

What does the future hold?

The implementation programme has been extended Trust-wide incorporating non-cancer patients. In particular, a model for care of dying stroke patients and patients who discontinue renal dialysis have been developed and successfully implemented. A care pathway for intensive care unit patients is currently under development.

In the hospice/specialist palliative care unit—Elaine Rosser

Why implement the LCP in the hospice setting?

Why do we need the LCP in the hospice setting when the care given is already excellent? The quality of the service is well recognized and care is delivered by a team of palliative care specialists. The value of the LCP lies in its ability to demonstrate measurable outcomes which provide evidence that we are delivering this high standard of care. The LCP is an excellent tool that identifies variances from normal practice. This provides us with a means to audit the reasons for the variance and change practice as required.

What does implementation of the LCP in the hospice setting involve?

The implementation of the LCP involves a clear understanding of the issues around change management (7). It is important that key people are assigned to the project.

They need be given the time and resources to move the project forward. One of their primary roles is to work with the team in a variety of ways to provide the support necessary for successful implementation of the LCP.

Education

It is of crucial importance that an ongoing education programme is put in place for all professionals involved in the project. When the LCP was being developed at the Marie Curie Centre Liverpool some of the staff were initially resistant to the LCP. They already had specialist knowledge and skills in palliative care and were documenting the care that they were giving, and could not see why they needed to use a pathway. However, following a series of meetings with staff it became evident that in some areas care was not always documented clearly and this could lead to confusion or lack of clarity. This can result in time being wasted in establishing a treatment plan for the patient. Discussion about the purpose, layout, and content of the LCP evoked lively debate. These discussions enabled us to focus on the roles of each professional and how these roles can sometimes overlap. This helped us to achieve a greater awareness of how we function as a team and highlighted the importance of team working and clear communication channels.

Pathway link nurse role

The Marie Curie Centre Liverpool seconded an experienced palliative care E grade staff nurse two days a week to focus on the project of implementing the LCP in the hospice setting. This role was crucial to the success of the project. This was because:

1. The postholder had a 'grass roots' understanding and 'strategic' knowledge of the value of the LCP to patient care.
2. The postholder had the clinical and managerial credibility to be able to challenge false views and champion concerns from staff that needed to be addressed.
3. The postholder had the time and resources to carry out the role successfully.

Initially, a series of open meetings were held for all staff to plan the time-scale for implementation of the LCP in the hospice. At a later stage structured meetings were held. Information packs and one-to-one group teaching sessions were made available to all staff.

A considerable amount of time was invested in establishing clear channels of communication. The importance of establishing this structure and the energy required to ensure the success of the project cannot be underestimated. The link nurse role remains of crucial importance in the Centre today. It has expanded to encompass the implementation of other pathways, for example, a Discharge pathway. It also now involves presenting at meetings and conferences and supporting pathway implementation across other Marie Curie centres.

Variance feedback

Whenever changes are introduced into an organization, feedback is necessary to demonstrate to staff how that change has benefited practice. Change can be exciting, but it is hard work and can be exhausting. Motivation needs to be continually stimulated. Regular feedback encourages this. The pathway link nurse held regular feedback sessions. They were received positively by all staff. The variance analysis was a useful means of auditing the care being given. It also provided evidence to support the need for change when this was challenged and assisted in the implementation of change when it was necessary.

Documentation

Initially fears and worries were expressed, particularly by nursing staff that the pathway format did not allow for the individuality of the patient or clinical decision making. However, when patient notes were reviewed, it was evident that much of the documentation relating to their care was repetitive, was not relevant or measurable, and was often disjointed.

Previously, it was an arduous task for the team caring for a patient to trawl through the records to ensure that they read all sections of the notes, i.e. nursing, allied health professions, social work, doctors, etc. There was a danger that if all the notes were not read, then an important element might be missed. The staff were encouraged to become involved in the design and structure of the documentation and became aware of the value of variance reporting. This led to a greater acceptance of the pathway. Today the hospice team would find it unacceptable not to utilize the LCP. The benefits have far outweighed the initial concerns.

What are the specific challenges of implementing the LCP in the hospice setting?

Managing change

The management of change is an ongoing process. It is important to plan and implement change carefully so that it is effective and efficient with positive outcomes (8).

Understanding of the LCP

Professionals in palliative care invest a considerable amount of time working outside the hospice providing education and support to other organizations. It is necessary to make it clear that patients who meet the criteria to go on an ICP may well come off the pathway if their condition improves.

Sharing of the LCP in other hospice/health care settings

It is important that the hospice takes a lead in supporting other areas for development of the LCP in their setting. The challenge to the hospice is to be able to provide the time and resources required for dissemination of the LCP outside of the hospice. The demands on the specialist team to provide their expertise are great.

The publication of the National cancer plan (5) and its implications for palliative care have increased the demand for expert consultancy as more and more organizations recognize the value care pathways as a means of measuring outcomes. Cancer Networks have now been established across the country and this national strategic approach to palliative care services has already resulted in the establishment of major education programmes on the LCP. For example, a district nurse education programme has been set up by the Merseyside and North Cheshire Cancer Network. The aim of this is to ensure that all staff gain a sound understanding of the purpose and value of the LCP and its role in improving care for dying patients.

What are the benefits for the hospice setting?

The LCP provides a formalized, structured tool which informs health care professionals when they are providing care of a high standard, but also highlights where there is room for improvement.

Example (a)

In the Marie Curie Centre Liverpool (MCCL) an audit was undertaken of the variances recorded on mouth care. This seemed to indicate that patients were not receiving mouth care at all. Following discussion with the nursing staff it became apparent that the patients were in fact receiving mouth care but that the wording and structure of this section of the pathway was ambiguous. The wording was subsequently modified and the ambiguity removed.

Example (b)

The LCP was expanded to include a section on Care After Death. This ensured that the patient's GP practice is always contacted to inform them of the patient's death. Prior to this there was no formalized documentation of this information and occasionally GPs were not informed of a patient's death. This was not acceptable.

Commissioning

The hospice works in partnership with the National Health Service which provides financial support for the services it gives (9, 10). It is important that the hospice is able to demonstrate how these services improve the quality of care for their patients (10). The LCP is an effective way to demonstrate these outcomes. The pathway analysis results provide useful evidence when requesting financial support due to increased dependency of patients. Prior to the LCP it was very difficult to provide evidence to back up such a request. The hospice knew it provided excellent care but had no way to demonstrate this.

In conclusion the LCP is an excellent research-based teaching tool for professionals and students who are not experienced in palliative care. Its structured approach allows for the holistic individual needs of each dying patient and ensures that all aspects of their care are addressed whether the needs of the patient are physical, psychosocial, emotional, or spiritual. It is an excellent tool that fits well into the clinical governance agenda (11, 12). It facilitates and fosters a culture of continual constructive challenge to clinical practice. How can we improve? What is working well? What is not? And what do we do about it? These questions are often asked and yet are not always fully addressed in a structured way. The pathway provides a clear way forward to do this.

The LCP is an excellent tool to benchmark Care of the Dying practices with other hospices and other settings. It encourages collaborative working practices with professionals and a sharing of practice developments that are research based.

In the community—Margaret Kendall

Why implement the LCP in the community?

There is nothing more satisfying to a community nurse than to provide best standard of care in someone's own home. Supplement this with enabling a dying patient to die at home in accordance with their wishes and Utopia is reached.

In reality however, this is not always be possible. This leads to feelings of frustration and inadequacy on the part of the health care professional, anguish to the patient, and guilt on the part of the carer.

All too often everything appears to be in place to care for a dying patient at home, but because of an escalation of symptoms, lack of knowledge and understanding on the part of the health care professional, or lack of communication between health care professional and carer, patients would be transferred in their final days or even hours of life to a hospice or hospital, leading to feelings of frustration and inadequacy.

The aim of implementing the Liverpool Care Pathway for the Dying Patient (LCP) in the Community was to provide a structure that could be used across the Community Trust to address these problems, as from discussions it became apparent that there was no measurable, equitable service being provided. The LCP provides a framework for care, which can be adapted to the individual patients' and carers' needs and wishes. By setting out the intended practice in the form of a document, the opportunity arises to provide measurable care that is clearly outcome based, but with the flexibility for adaptation.

A base review undertaken prior to using the pathway highlighted that interventions were being undertaken which were unnecessary and there were areas of educational deficit that needed to be addressed by a programme of education.

The initial assessment of the patient prior to inclusion on the LCP follows the same criteria used within both the hospice and hospital settings. Because of the different setting, i.e. the patients' home, some of the goals on the other pathways were not applicable necessitating minor adaptation.

It was hoped that by implementing the LCP in the community, problems could be anticipated, and suitable solutions prepared pre-emptively, and the nursing staff would have a measure of satisfaction at the standard of care being achieved.

What does implementation of the LCP into the community involve?

The former North Mersey Community Trust is an area with diverse social, economic, ethnic, and cultural strata. Some areas have very high unemployment, social deprivation, and drug problems. Other areas are extremely affluent with highly educated inhabitants. The only thing they appeared to have in common was that a cohort among their inhabitants would die of cancer.

The first problem we encountered was to set up a working party to examine the feasibility of initiating such a concept into the community. Only a handful of like-minded people felt they could set aside enough time to work on the project. A core team of four people examined the concept in more depth, familiarized themselves with the documentation, and set out an action plan to take forward what would undoubtedly be a huge project.

It was decided that the implementation would take place slowly, to lessen the possibility of failure of the project. Nevertheless there was an unexpected degree of cynicism when discussions first took place. There was a feeling among many of the nursing staff that this would prove to be yet another 'paper exercise', with extra work for them with no positive outcomes. It was necessary to have three separate discussion sessions, with all staff concerned, when the original document was redrafted for community use.

Among many of the interesting discussions that took place was one around the title of the document itself. Some staff felt uncomfortable that the word 'dying' was included in the script, bringing into question whether the staff themselves had issues with the fact of death, and they found this difficult to cope with, not the title of the document itself.

Base review

Before any new way of working could be implemented a base review to obtain a picture of the current situation was undertaken. Six sets of case sheets of patients who had recently died at home from cancer, were requested from each locality in North Mersey. This gave 36 sets of notes to review.

In spite of the staff in the localities all being briefed on the project, and knowing what we were undertaking there was an air of suspicion. Why did we want the notes? What were we looking for? Were we checking up on the nurses?

We also examined the corresponding notes in the GP surgery but found that in the majority of cases, not only could we not decipher the writing, but also there was very little supporting evidence that we could use for review.

The results of the base review were illuminating. Whilst we knew the nurses had provided a very high standard of care for the dying person, there was little evidence to support the care given in the notes. According to the ethicist John Tingle, 'in a court of law if the evidence is not written; it is deemed that it has not been done'. Regular systematic review of symptoms appeared to be sporadic. The results are detailed in Figure 8.1.

- 83% of cases (n = 30) examined showed that there was written evidence that analgesia had been prescribed.
- 56% of patients (n = 20) were prescribed an anticholinergic.
- 61% of cases (n = 21) were prescribed a sedative.
- 56% of cases (n = 20) were prescribed an anti-emetic.
- Documented evidence that discussion had taken place with the relatives on what to do after a death was not easily obtained.
- No evidence could be obtained from the notes that any assessment of non-essential medication had taken place.
- Little evidence was found that communication had taken place or was meaningful. When examining the participation by patient, family, and friends in the decision making process evidence from the review showed that this participation was only documented in 17% of cases among patients, and 37% among relatives.

Figure 8.1 Results of the base review.

Feeding back the results of the base review required huge amounts of diplomacy to allay the anxiety of the staff at this point. We were clear to reinforce that the evidence from this base review was not unusual, and whilst we were confident that the care had been undertaken, we were seeking written evidence to support the facts.

Pilot project

The next part of the process was to compile all the evidence from the base review into a presentation, with an outline of the project to prepare staff for pilot project.

It had previously been agreed that the documentation used in the hospital setting should be replicated for community use. The only changes made were to parts of the pathway, which clearly were pertinent to acute sector only, e.g. resuscitation status, collection of belongings after death, collection of certificates from general office, etc. These parts were deleted and appropriate interventions pertinent to the community inserted.

It was decided that the document and implementation of the LCP should be piloted in two very different general practice settings. One practice consisted of five GPs, already proactive in palliative care, with a good supportive primary health care team. Patient mix was varied as the practice had two surgeries, one in a socially deprived area with high rates of unemployment, and the other in a new estate with low rates of unemployment and generally inhabited by professionals and affluent families. The other pilot site was a single-handed GP practice in an inner city area. Staffing levels in the PHCT were often poor, due to sickness and unavailability of staff. The patient population was a mix of elderly patients, and a large ethnic minority population.

Staff in the practice were given additional training and education on the project, and extra support was given to the PHCT. Collaborative visits with nurses to dying patients on the LCP were given by the project team, in order to ensure problems were not arising due to misinterpretation. After a few initial hiccoughs this worked well.

Initially it was envisaged the pilot would run for three months in each practice. However, numbers of patients fitting the criteria to be entered on the LCP were slow to recruit, the project was therefore extended for another three months in order to give a more meaningful evaluation. After six months, 16 patients, all dying of cancer, had been placed on the pathway. Mean time on the pathway was three days, with a range of three hours to ten days. The numbers of episodes of pain and agitation were analysed and the results demonstrated:

(a) The documentation was more comprehensive.

(b) The nurses achieved a high level of satisfaction at the care they were able to give.

(c) No patients were transferred from their chosen place of death.

Problems highlighted were the delay in obtaining vital equipment, and the lack of ability to obtain necessary medications out of hours. This latter point only arose on one occasion and was in fact due to the proactive prescribing of medication not taking place.

Analysis of the data from the pathways was undertaken by the audit department of the Trust, and was presented back to the pilot practice. A comparison with the pre-pathway data from the pilot practices showed that the implementation of the LCP made a measurable difference to the documented care of patients dying at home.

Post-implementation audit showed that the level of documented evidence had risen dramatically.

Wider implementation

Following this successful pilot study it was agreed that the project should be implemented on a Trust-wide basis. Because of the number of GP practices within the Trust, approximately 130 at the time of the implementation, a process had to be devised to roll the programme out. Letters were sent to each practice, outlining the project, and containing the results of the pilot study. Practices were asked to self-nominate to take the project forward in the first wave. Forty practices nominated themselves, and by chance the spread across the area was good. The Community Macmillan Clinical Nurse Specialists working in each area agreed to be key people to assist their own practices, in conjunction with the district nurses.

Education programme

A rolling programme of education was provided for all members of the PHCT involved in the second wave. Staff were familiarized with the documentation. The educational programme also involved the following:

Education programme

Pain control.

Management of nausea and vomiting.

Management of constipation.

Communication skills.

Dealing with collusion.

Dealing with loss and bereavement.

Psychological issues around caring for dying patients.

How nurses deal with loss and grief.

Management of syringe drivers.

Breaking bad news.

Handling difficult questions.

Ethical issues in palliative care.

This programme was delivered by the Macmillan Community Clinical Nurse specialist team on an ongoing basis. It was delivered as a two-day course with workshops, case studies, and self-directed study as an integral part of the day.

Additional support was given to nurses when they initially cared for a patient who fitted the criteria for pathway inclusion.

Refresher sessions had to be held for some staff that attended the initial training, but then had no patients who fitted the criteria for some time and had forgotten something of the process. Pathway updates were included on the education programme provided by the Macmillan CNS team in order to keep the LCP high profile.

This same process was undertaken for two further cohorts of interested practices. The remaining practices that had not put themselves forward to undertake the project were also contacted. Trying to implement the LCP in these practices was problematic. Eventually the project was implemented across the entire Trust, although with antagonism in some areas.

What are the specific challenges of implementing the LCP into the community?

The initial problem was one of suspicion when undertaking the base review as previously recounted. Other problems varied from outright hostility of some staff that the way they were delivering care should be examined, to feelings that this was a paper exercise and would not make a difference. Sadly some of the antagonism remains to date and a very small number of nurses refuse to fill in the documentation. The LCP project is still in place three years later, with a real difference being made to care of patients dying at home with close communication being undertaken with the carers.

What are the benefits for the community setting?

Variances from the pathway were analysed in batches of 10 by the Trust audit department and the data collated. After a six month period of wide implementation 86 patients had been cared for using the LCP.

The results are as shown in Figure 8.2. These show a considerable improvement from the initial base review results shown in Figure 8.1.

Case history

Mrs A was a 56-year-old lady who had been diagnosed in 1997 as having a Pancoast tumour of her right lung. Her initial treatment of radiotherapy had proven to be successful in that she was relatively symptom free for a period of nine months with only minimal medication.

Unfortunately in early 1998 she developed symptoms of superior vena cava obstruction. This necessitated the use of high dose corticosteroids followed by further radiotherapy. Sadly her condition relapsed within two months when it was decided that no

- 93% (n = 80) had their drugs converted to a subcutaneous route as a matter of routine.
- 91% (n = 78) were routinely prescribed anti-cholinergics and anti-emetics.
- 96% of patients (n = 83) were written up for sedation.
- Documented evidence that discussion around the plan of care had been undertaken was seen in 88% of cases (n = 76).

Figure 8.2 Results after wide implementation.

further active treatment was possible and she was kept comfortable at home with active symptom control.

On two occasions she had to be taken to hospital at the weekend as an emergency admission, when perhaps with forward planning this could have been avoided. Referral to the Macmillan Clinical Nurse Specialist took place after the second admission and a joint visit was undertaken with the district nursing care manager to the patient's home. Assessment of the needs of Mrs A and her family took place. Following the guidelines set out in the LCP it was decided that a supply of the most commonly used drugs should be made available in Mrs As home. The GPs written permission to give them was sought, should the nursing staff deem it to be necessary. A supply of diamorphine, hyoscine hydrobromide, and midazolam was obtained, together with a syringe driver for subcutaneous administration of the drugs.

These supplies remained untouched in the patient's home for 15 days. The family and Mrs A all expressed a feeling of reassurance from knowing that they were there, and that Mrs A could hopefully achieve her wish to die at home without another admission to hospital.

On the afternoon of the 16th day Mrs As condition deteriorated. She complained of feeling extremely dyspnoeic, and had developed marked oedema in her face and upper thorax. Following telephone discussion with her GP, the district nurse set up the syringe driver containing a small quantity of diamorphine and hyoscine. The GP visited later and found Mrs A to be settling comfortably, with no obvious distress. She roused slightly during the evening and complained that she was getting some chest pain, but said she could cope with that but was frightened because she realized that she was dying. The night district nursing team were contacted, and called to give a subcutaneous injection of midazalom and diamorphine.

Mrs A spent a comfortable night, and roused again soon after dawn. She was not in pain and was calm. She asked her family to open the curtains so she could see the sun coming up. Having expressed delight at the fact that it was going to be a sunny day she closed her eyes and died peacefully with her family around her.

It is my belief that without this forward planning afforded by the LCP, and by pre-empting problems, Mrs A and her family could not have achieved their longed for wishes.

Conclusions

In conclusion although very time-consuming initially and fraught with administrative difficulties the project was a very worthy one. With hindsight a larger full-time project team would have been useful as the majority of the work was done by myself and a pathway co-ordinator, who was also working on other projects. Without the support of my CNS colleagues I would have been unable to undertake this work. One of the most time-consuming parts of the project was the education both pre- and during implementation. This has been quantified as around 72 hours for cross Trust implementation. This element alone should not be underestimated in time or intensity.

Ongoing analysis of the variances shows that the level of documented evidence of care has increased dramatically. Proactive prescribing of medication is now the norm. There is strong evidence of good communication between families and the staff caring for them. Patients and carers wishes are taken into account. Unnecessary interventions have ceased. Equity of care can be demonstrated. Staff have written evidence to highlight problems. Evidence from the variances has been used to change procedures and practice for availability and delivery of vital equipment. Difficult case scenarios have been resolved by collaborative working. Crisis admission to hospital in the dying phase is reduced and in many cases totally eliminated, as both medical and nursing staff have increased confidence in looking after dying patients.

Feedback was given to staff at locality meetings and a six monthly written review was planned to incorporate all the variances that had been highlighted in that same period.

Initially the implementation of the LCP was for patients dying of cancer, but its use has now been extended to encompass the care of all patients dying at home. The reality of its impact was highlighted in a letter received from the widow of a patient who had renal failure. She stated:-

"Because my husband had been ill for so long I always knew what dialysis and blood tests were due on which day. When he came home to die I felt that there was no longer a plan. When the nurse came and talked to us about the pathway I knew this was what we were missing. While we didn't know how long .... would live, at least we knew that everything was being taken into account. This made so much difference to the two of us."

This says it all!

In the nursing home setting— Kim Barrow

Why implement the LCP in the nursing home setting?

Many nursing homes provide an excellent standard of care to patients, particularly those who are dying. In the past it has not been possible to prove this fact. As a nursing home matron, I often felt that the care given in the nursing home environment was considered by many to be inferior to that given in other settings. The Liverpool Integrated Care Pathway (LCP) provides proof of the high standard of care being given.

What does implementation of the LCP in the nursing home setting involve?

Before implementing the LCP, it was necessary to carry out a base review using data from the records of past patients. The base review confirmed that the care being given was of a high standard and that the patients had died peacefully. However, this was not being adequately documented. With the full support of the palliative care consultant and local Macmillan nurse the LCP was introduced by the following means:

(a) Education of staff relating to the document itself.

(b) Explanation to staff as to the benefits of the document and the impact it would have to patient care documentation.

(c) Discussion with GPs involved in the care of our palliative patients.

A direct link was established between the nursing home, the research assistant, and the consultant so that the data from our LCP could be analysed and fed back to the unit. The implementation of the LCP was quite straightforward. The unit was small and therefore the bureaucracy very limited. The document was simply implemented.

What are the specific challenges of implementing the LCP in the nursing home setting?

One difficulty we did encounter was with the introduction of the LCP to the GPs in the community. Many GPs have little contact with dying patients on a daily basis and may only care for one or two patients a year. They are often unfamiliar with protocols for symptom control. This is compounded by the use of the out of hours service. Doctors providing this service are often seeing the patient for the first time and are reluctant to prescribe the use of a syringe driver and the drugs required for effective symptom control. The first cohort of the LCP to be analysed demonstrated from the variance analysis that:

(a) GP refused to prescribe medication in line with protocol.

(b) Out of hours service refused to prescribe medication.

(c) Medication not available out of hours at local pharmacies.

It was clear from these findings it was going to be important to work with GPs and with the local pharmacy to overcome these problems. With great difficulty, meetings with all the local GP practices were arranged to discuss the LCP and the analysed data. Many of the GPs expressed concerns regarding the prescription of medication on a sliding scale and in advance of use. It was agreed that a trial using the next three appropriate patients should be undertaken before reviewing the situation.

The local supply pharmacist was also contacted and the difficulties were explained. It was agreed the drugs required by the protocol within the LCP would be stocked and also an emergency contact system would be arranged. The trial with three patients was very successful and it was possible to positively review the practices developed with the GPs involved.

What are the benefits for the nursing home setting?

Forward planning is of the utmost importance in the nursing home setting. In this environment there is not the luxury of an on-site doctor or stock medications. It is therefore necessary for the staff to be proactive. This is something that the LCP encourages. It is vital that medication is prescribed as soon as it is assessed as necessary so that it can be obtained quickly and be on-site ready for use. It is important to establish a relationship of trust with the prescribing GP. To build such a relationship takes time and it was policy in the nursing home that no syringe driver should be commenced without consultation with myself as the specialist practitioner. Nursing staff felt more comfortable with this and the GPs felt that this gave them more confidence in prescribing proactively. The GPs also liaised with the out of hours service if the patient was expected to die, so that the doctor on duty would be aware of the treatment protocol. This proved to be very successful.

The profile of the nursing home increased dramatically over a two year period and we were receiving referrals for some very complex cases. The LCP had enabled us to care effectively for complex symptoms and we were able to prove this fact. Staff within the home find the document invaluable. It is easy to use, less time-consuming than the Kardex system, and enables staff to effectively treat the patients in their care. Many staff commented that they found the document useful in teaching other professionals and carers. The LCP became part of the induction training for all new staff. After a period of approximately three years, the local GP practices started to send the GP registrars to the home to be educated in how to use the LCP. We have also taught Pharmacy students.

Nursing students had been regular attendees at the home prior to the implementation of the LCP. Following its implementation we were able to offer more effective teaching and the comments received on evaluation documents were extremely positive with regard to the learning experience. In summary the implementation of the LCP in the nursing home environment requires:

◆ Determination.

◆ Belief.

◆ Patience.

◆ Team building.

◆ Proactive planning.

◆ Collaboration.

It is not easy to implement any change. Often it is a long and hard struggle, but one which is well worth the effort involved. The benefits by far outweigh the difficulties and the most important outcome is that quality of care can be proven and deficits identified and acted on.

Outcomes of implementing the LCP:

◆ Proof of best practice.

◆ Holistic documentation.

◆ Multi-professional recognition.

◆ Trained staff recruitment and retention.

◆ Improved staff morale.

Knowing that you do a good job and being able to prove it are two different things. The LCP facilitates the achievement of both aims. Staff were empowered by the use of the LCP. The care given was research based and provided legal protection, in that the practices undertaken were considered and proved to be best practice. Patient care was regularly evaluated and symptoms where possible proactively treated.

It should be remembered that the LCP is not written in stone and can be amended to suit specific site requirements. The protocols in the nursing home setting are different from those in all other localities and the LCP was altered to encompass these differences. Assessment and after death formalities were altered to facilitate the needs of the unit and the protocols set down by the registering authority. Undoubtedly the nursing home's profile has improved as a result of the LCP. Prior to the LCP, nursing home staff often felt like second class professionals working in an environment that had been criticized for many years. The implementation of the LCP has increased staff confidence, self-esteem, and credibility with other professionals.

In conclusion the LCP proved that a small nursing home could provide effective care to those who are dying and to their families. The difficulties of caring for the dying in the nursing home environment are complex and should not be underestimated by other professionals. It is an environment that is nurse led. There are no on-site facilities if a patient deteriorates and nursing staff have to be competent and active in forward planning the care of their patients. They need to have a broad knowledge and to be skilled in the assessment of a patient and in the risk assessment of potential emergency situations and to be fully aware of the procedures to be undertaken. In this environment nurses are the prime professionals responsible for the safe delivery of care. It is often the case that the nursing staff is more knowledgeable than the medical staff with regard to the palliative care needs of the patients and the medications required. This is a result of nurses giving care on a daily basis. Medical staff do not do this. Nurses in the nursing home need to be assertive and it is important to support their practices. Supporting documentation was made available for nurses to utilize if there were any differences in opinion as to the best protocol for care.

If patients are unable to die at home for whatever reason the nursing home environment can provide care in a home style surrounding. This should not be undervalued. Nursing homes can provide a unique environment for patients and their relatives at a time of grief and stress and the importance of this should not be underestimated. In turn nursing homes must provide 'best practice' care based on current research. Managers and owners of homes must encourage learning and development not only for qualified nurses but for all staff. Care assistants are major contributors to care in this environment and their contribution should not be undervalued. Nursing homes can provide care equal to that of any other establishment of care. NOW WE CAN PROVE IT!

References

1. ONS Office of National Statistics. (2000). http://www.statistics.gov.uk
2. Ahmedzai, S. (1982). Dying in hospital: the residents' viewpoint. *Br. Med. J.*, **285**, 712–4.
3. Department of Social Security. (1997). *What to do after a death.* Department of Social Security (September).
4. Murphy, D. (2001). *The Liverpool Care Pathway for the Dying Patient.* NHS Trusts Commissioners' Guide.
5. Department of Health. (2000). *The NHS cancer plan.* Department of Health, London (September).
6. Hutchison, T. and Kelly, A. (2000). Raising the profile of palliative care in acute hospital wards. *Macmillan Voice*, **16**, 5.
7. Paton, R. A. and McCalman, J. (2000). *Change management: A guide to effective implementation.* Sage Publications Ltd.
8. Belbin, R. M. (1981). *Management teams: Why they succeed or fail.* Butterworth–Heinemann.
9. NCHSPCS. (1999). *Palliative care 2000: Commissioning through partnership.* National Council for Hospice and Specialist Palliative Care Services (March).

10. **NCHSPCS.** (1999). *The definition and measurement of quality in palliative care: Briefing number 3.* National Council for Hospice and Specialist Palliative Care Services (December).

11. **Department of Health.** (1997). *The new NHS modem, dependable.* Department of Health (December).

12. **NCHSPCS.** (1999). *Clinical governance: Briefing number 2.* National Council for Hospice and Specialist Palliative Care Services (November).

Chapter 9

Evaluating the Liverpool Care Pathway for the Dying Patient (LCP) and future developments

John Ellershaw and Susie Wilkinson

The initial aim of developing the LCP was to transfer best practice from the hospice setting to other health care settings. The development, implementation, and dissemination of the project has led to over 100 palliative care services in the UK undergoing training to implement the LCP. An important aspect of implementing the LCP is the analysis and feedback of data recorded. This will be discussed in this chapter.

During this development phase interesting questions have been asked which will also be addressed including:

(a) Can the LCP be used for non-cancer patients?

(b) Can integrated care pathways be developed for other aspects of palliative care?

(c) Has the LCP a role in research and development?

Analysis and feedback of data from the LCP

There are a number of ways that data from the LCP can be analysed and collated to set standards and inform best practice. Analysis of individual variances has the potential to highlight issues that can then be addressed. For example:

(a) Educational issues, e.g. issues of hydration or prescribing in the dying phase.

(b) Resource issues, e.g. lack of specialist mattresses.

(c) Modifications that would improve the LCP, e.g. altering prompts.

It is also possible to collate data from the three sections of the LCP. For initial assessment the goals are recorded as:

◆ Yes

◆ No (variance)

Figure 9.1 is an example of results from the LCP. It shows that overall the unit is achieving 80–100% of 'achieved' goals in all except goal 9, which is communication with the primary health care team.

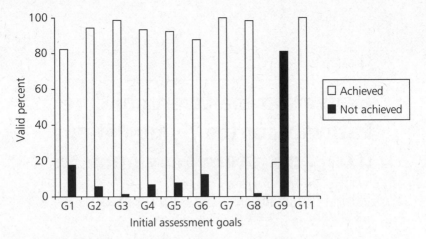

Figure 9.1 Achieved and not achieved (variance) initial assessment goals: (valid %).

Ongoing care is assessed as either:

♦ Achieved

♦ Variance

Figure 9.2 is an example of the variance recordings for pain, respiratory tract secretions, and agitation. It illustrates that 52% of patients had no pain variances in the last 48 hours of life, i.e. no pain in the dying phase. Nine percent had three or more pain variances which can be reviewed to identify the causes. These variances may have been unavoidable but may identify avoidable variances such as the availability of drugs.

Symptoms	Number of variances (%)			
	0	1	2	3 or more
Pain	52%	31%	8%	9%
Agitation	49%	31%	16%	4%
Chest secretions	59%	25%	13%	3%

Figure 9.2 Analysis of variances in the last 48 hours of life.

Care after death is recorded as either:

♦ Yes

♦ No (variance)

Figure 9.3 is an example of the results that can be collated from the care after death section of the LCP.

It is possible using the information analysed from the LCP to contribute to audit in a unit by looking at outliers which will inform case audit, but also by doing comparative audit from year to year to see any trends in the delivery of care. It may also be possible to do a comparison between units although care must be taken to ensure that

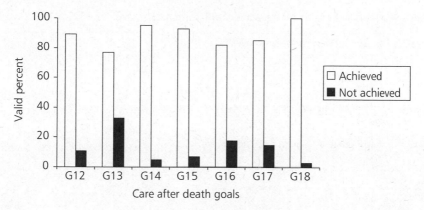

Figure 9.3 Achieved and not achieved (variance) care after death goals: (valid %).

the samples are from a similar population. In the future this may lead to the development of national performance indicators for care of the dying.

In 1997 clinical governance was formally introduced as a concept in the NHS with the publication of the white paper *The new NHS modern dependable* (1). This document emphasizes for the first time the importance of the quality of clinical care. The objective of clinical governance is to ensure that the patient receives the best quality of care throughout their journey and to learn from patient experiences in order to provide services that better meet patient need. The LCP is one tool that can help to meet the requirements of the clinical governance agenda, providing demonstrable standards and outcomes of care for patients. The LCP project is currently incorporated in the Cancer Collaborative project in the Merseyside and North Cheshire Cancer Network.

Can the LCP be used for non-cancer patients?

The LCP was originally developed for use with cancer patients and therefore the criteria for entry onto the pathway are appropriate for this population. However, it must be restated that the most important criteria for entry onto the LCP is that the multidisciplinary team are in agreement that the patient is entering the dying phase and has only hours/days to live. Experience of using the LCP has extended to non-cancer patients including those with chronic obstructive airways disease, stroke patients, cardiac failure, intensive care unit, and renal failure patients. In each of these disease-specific categories, different issues arise regarding diagnosing dying and applying appropriate criteria. In most cases little change is needed to the LCP, however, for some specific situations, for example patients discontinuing renal dialysis, a more explicit initial entry criteria has been developed Table 9.1.

Although some modification may be required for the initial criteria for commencing the LCP, the goals of care have not been changed within disease categories. Again, changes and modifications of the prompts for the goals have been undertaken in order to personalize the document for the appropriate department. The same intensive education process is required to implement the LCP successfully. This wider dissemination of the LCP into the non-cancer population is an important step forward to disseminating best practice for palliative care to this population and has been welcomed by health care professionals when it has been introduced.

Table 9.1 Modified criteria for initiation of LCP for renal patients

Goal	Reason for stopping dialysis is clear	
	Not tolerating dialysis	Deterioration in spite of dialysis
	Patient's wishes	Patient unconscious
	Other	
Goal	Patient and family members aware of why dialysis is being discontinued	
	Yes	No
Goal	Appropriate placement for ongoing care	
	Yes	No

Can integrated care pathways be developed for other aspects of palliative care?

Following introduction of the LCP into the Marie Curie Centre Liverpool and the Royal Liverpool University Hospitals further consideration was undertaken regarding development of integrated care pathways to improve patient care and multidisciplinary communication. One area highlighted by staff was the discharge home of patients from the hospice to community and in particular the rapid discharge to home for patients wishing to die at home from the hospital to the community. This work was particularly important as it included improving communication between the secondary and primary care interface.

The hospice discharge pathway

The hospice discharge pathway was developed with members of the hospice and community teams. Prior to developing the discharge pathway there were a number of documents held by each individual group including medical, nursing, occupational therapist, physiotherapist, and social worker which were not combined. There was duplication of information and only verbal transfer of information between disciplines. The development of the discharge pathway has lead to one document being used by all disciplines. This records key events of the patient's admission together with the planning for discharge, the planned care following discharge including follow-up and details of the patient's drugs, together with their indications and times to be taken. The new discharge pathway has streamlined the process of discharge planning and has proved popular with all disciplines. It has also lead to the patient taking a copy of the discharge pathway home and therefore a patient held record of admission and discharge from the hospice is available in the patient's home to be accessed by the primary health care team. Again, this has improved communication between secondary and primary care and has been well received in the community.

The rapid discharge home from hospital for dying patients

The specialist hospital palliative care team at the Royal Liverpool University Hospitals identified the scenario of a patient who is entering the dying phase who expresses a wish to die at home. Logistically, if dying patients in hospital express a wish to die at home this is often perceived as an unmanageable crisis. This can be due to factors such as:

(a) The short length of time available to organize maximum home care services.

(b) Ensuring that the patients and families best interests are fulfilled safely and effectively.

(c) Ensuring availability of appropriate drugs.

(d) Guidelines for ambulance staff in case the patient dies during the transfer home.

(e) Clear lines of communication between hospital and community teams.

The rapid discharge home pathway aims to change this into a manageable episode, pre-emptively preparing for the patients expected deterioration at home.

This planning requires a multi-agency approach and community and hospital need to work closely together. A multidisciplinary group was convened with representation from the hospital and community, to develop an integrated care pathway for rapid discharge home for dying patients. The implementation of the rapid discharge pathway has streamlined the process of transferring a patient home from days to a matter of hours and has been successfully implemented at the Royal Liverpool University Hospitals. This pathway ultimately enables patients dying in hospital to have choice over where they die (2).

Integrated care pathways probably offer the best opportunity within palliative care to develop multidisciplinary notes. Integrated care pathways can facilitate cross boundary working and documentation. We are currently piloting a project where patients who are seen in the out-patient department in hospital have the same documentation as those being seen in the hospice. This means that if the patients are then followed up in the hospice the same notes can be incorporated instead of rewriting the whole history. This facilitation of closely working together across boundaries leads to a more integrated service for patients and more effective communication and time utilization for palliative care professionals.

Has the LCP a role in research and development?

Palliative care research is very much in its infancy. For example, unlike other specialities in medicine up until 1997 only 11 randomized controlled trials related to palliative care had been published most of which focused on pain control (3).

There has been a dearth of studies evaluating the management of other common symptoms (such as nausea, vomiting, constipation, terminal restless, and psychological distress) or service provision, although the need for practice to be based on reliable evidence rather than anecdote has been recognized since the foundation of the modern hospice movement. Much of the research undertaken to date has been limited and fragmented, with small scale single centre, descriptive studies being the norm. There are a number of explanations for this relative lack of palliative care research:

1. Research training related to palliative care has not traditionally been an integrated part of nursing or medical education.

2. Palliative care services over the last decade have developed so rapidly that meeting the clinical needs of patients and their families has tended to take priority over the need to establish a sound evidence base.

3. There are perceived ethical and practical difficulties in undertaking research with patients with a poor prognosis. Attrition rates are high.

4. Outcome measures for palliative care patients differ from other patient groups.

The LCP records the key outcomes of care and the efficacy of symptom control. In this way the LCP has the potential to develop the evidence base for the care of the dying. For example, data has been collected by using the LCP at the Marie Curie Centre Liverpool. From the analysis of this data it has been possible to describe the pattern of symptom control regarding pain, agitation, and respiratory tract secretions in the last 48 hours of life (4). It is also possible to use the LCP to look at new innovations or developments. For example, the introduction of the fentanyl patch for pain relief in cancer lead to some confusion about analgesic control in the dying phase, whether to continue the patch or discontinue it. We have been able to demonstrate using the LCP that continuing the fentanyl patch does not compromise pain control in the dying phase (5). Similarly introduction of new drugs for agitation or respiratory tract secretions could be compared with current standard practice.

Teaching and education

The use of the LCP as an educational tool has already been highlighted. It is an effective way of demonstrating and articulating clearly how dying patients are cared for and can be utilized in undergraduate teaching for the health care professional who will come into contact with dying patients as well as incorporating it into postgraduate education. It has been valued in situations where new staff have joined existing teams, for example, in hospices as it clearly outlines the process of care.

Future developments

The electronic health record

The Electronic Health Record (HER) and the Electronic Patient Record (EPR). Electronic development of care pathways is set out in the IM&T Strategy which was published in 1998. It is identified at level three of the EPR and a number of organizations are currently piloting electronic pathways with some success.

The principle of developing paper-based pathways initially seems to be still accepted because of the culture changes required with multidisciplinary teamwork and a unified patient document. However, these are exciting times and the opportunities to combine conditions, include alerts, insert guidance, and support clinical decisions within an electronic format is something many health care professions look forward to with impatience. The groundwork which has been done over the last ten years will not be wasted as new electronic systems are developed and implemented. Whatever the future of the health service in the UK, it is certain that Care Pathways will be a predominantly contributing factor.

The educational challenge of diagnosing dying

The LCP was developed to specifically address the issues of patients dying distressing deaths, i.e. in pain or agitation in acute hospitals and to relieve the distress of relatives who were unsupported in this dying phase. The introduction of the LCP has greatly improved symptom control for patients and support for relatives and there is an interesting shift of emphasis in the health care professionals in the hospital to raising the question regarding how to diagnose dying more clearly. It would appear that once a formal process for care of the dying is put in place then health care professionals recognize the importance of delivering optimum care in this phase. Empowerment and awareness at this level raises the issue that patients should not be deprived of the best care and therefore being able to accurately know when the patients are entering the dying phase is important. This leads to a refocusing of the education programme and also the need to develop an evidence base regarding this important issue.

A European perspective

Work is currently ongoing with a research team based in Rotterdam at the cancer centre and in a palliative care unit in a nursing home which has lead to the translation of the pathway into Dutch. This has followed rigorous criteria as outlined by the EORTC for translating to different languages (6). Initial implementation and analysis have been favourable and ongoing work is currently being undertaken regarding its development and dissemination. The potential development of this work with clinical indicators for dying patients across Europe is an exciting prospect.

References

1. **Department of Health.** (1997). *The new NHS modem, dependable.* Department of Health (December).
2. **Foster, A.** (2002). *Development of a care pathway for rapid discharge for patients who wish to die at home.* Macmillan National Institute of Education, Conference proceedings, pp. 37–9.
3. **Rinck, G. C., van den Bos, G. A., de Haes, J., Schade, E., and Veenhof, C. H.** (1997). Methodological issues in effectiveness research on palliative cancer care: A systematic review. *J. Clin. Oncol.*, 15(4), 1697–707.
4. **Ellershaw, J. E., Smith, C., Overill, S., Walker, S. E., and Aldridge, J.** (2001). Care of the dying: Setting standards for symptom control in the last 48 hours of life. *J. Pain Symptom Manage.*, 21(1), 12–7.
5. **Ellershaw, J. E., Kinder, C., Aldridge, J., Allison, M., and Smith, J. C.** (2002). Care of the dying: Is pain control compromised or enhanced by continuation of the fentanyl transdermal patch in the dying phase? *J. Pain Symptom Manage.*, 24(4), 398–403.
6. **Cull, A., Sprangers, M., Bjordal, K., and Aaronson, N.** (1998). *EORTC quality of life study group translation procedure.* EORTC Quality of Life Study Group.

Appendix 1

LCP—Hospital

NAME: .... UNIT NO: ....

The Royal Liverpool University Hospitals – Broadgreen and Liverpool NHS Trust

THE LIVERPOOL INTEGRATED CARE PATHWAY FOR THE TERMINAL/DYING PHASE

A Care Pathway is intended as a guide to treatment and an aid to documenting patient progress. Of course, practitioners are free to exercise their own professional judgement, however any alteration to the practice identified within this ICP must be noted as a variance on the sheet at the back of the pathway.

*Reference: Changing Gear – Guidelines for Managing the Last Days of Life in Adults. National Council for Hospice and Specialist Palliative Care Services. Northamptonshire: Land & Unwin (Data Sciences) Ltd, 1997

CONSULTANT: **NAMED NURSE:**   **WARD:**

INSTRUCTIONS FOR USE

1. All goals are in **heavy** typeface. Interventions, which act as prompts to support the goals, are in normal type.

2. If a goal is not achieved (i.e. variance) then chart on the variance section on the back page.

3. The Palliative Care guidelines are printed on the pages at the end of the pathway. Please make reference as necessary.

4. If you have any problems regarding the Pathway contact the Palliative Care Team.

ALL PERSONNEL COMPLETING THE CARE PATHWAY PLEASE SIGN BELOW

Name (Print)	Full Signature	Initials	Professional Title	Date

CRITERIA FOR ICP – DO NOT PUT ON THE PATHWAY UNLESS

The Multidisciplinary team have agreed the patient is dying and two of the following apply:-

The patient is bedbound   ❏   Semi-Comatose   ❏

Only able to take sips of fluids   ❏   No longer able to take tablets   ❏

IF YOU HAVE ANY PROBLEMS

PLEASE

CONTACT THE PALLIATIVE

CARE TEAM

INTEGRATED CARE PATHWAY FOR THE TERMINAL/DYING PHASE

NAME: .... UNIT NO: .... DATE: ....

SECTION 1	PATIENT ASSESSMENT			
DIAGNOSIS	PRIMARY SECONDARY Date of In-patient admission .... Ethnicity ....……..			
PHYSICAL CONDITION	Unable to swallow Yes ❏ No ❏ Nausea Yes ❏ No ❏ Vomiting Yes ❏ No ❏ Constipated Yes ❏ No ❏ Confused Yes ❏ No ❏ Agitation Yes ❏ No ❏ Restless Yes ❏ No ❏ Distressed Yes ❏ No ❏		Aware Yes ❏ No ❏ Conscious Yes ❏ No ❏ UTI Problems Yes ❏ No ❏ Catheterised Yes ❏ No ❏ Respiratory Tract Secretions Yes ❏ No ❏ Dyspnoea Yes ❏ No ❏ Pain Yes ❏ No ❏ Other Yes ❏ No ❏	

COMFORT MEASURES	(If 'No' chart as variance on the back page)
	
	Goal 1: Current medication assessed and non essentials discontinued Yes ❏ No ❏
	          Appropriate oral drugs converted to subcutaneous route and syringe
	          driver commenced if appropriate
	          Inappropriate medication discontinued			

Goal 2: PRN subcutaneous medication written up for list below as per Protocol Yes ❏ No ❏	
(see blue sheets at back of ICP for guidance)	
Pain	Analgesia
Nausea & Vomiting	Anti–emetic
Agitation	Sedative
Respiratory Tract Secretions	Anticholinergic

Goal 3: Discontinue inappropriate interventions   Yes ❏   No ❏
     Blood Test
     Antibiotics
     I.V.'s (fluids/medications)
     Not for Cardiopulmonary Resuscitation (Please record below)

Doctor's signature ....…........   Date ....

Goal 3a: Decisions to discontinue inappropriate nursing interventions taken   Yes ❏   No ❏
         Routine Turning Regime (turn for comfort only)
         Taking Vital signs

Goal 3b: Syringe driver set up within 4 hours of Doctors order   Yes ❏   No ❏   N/A ❏

Nurse signature ....   Date ....   Time ....

INTEGRATED CARE PATHWAY FOR THE TERMINAL/DYING PHASE

NAME.. UNIT NO: .... DATE: ....

SECTION 1	Patient assessment Contd/
PSYCHOLOGICAL/ INSIGHT	**Goal 4: Ability to communicate in English assessed as adequate** Yes ❑ No ❑ (See Hospital translation policy)

		Comatosed	Yes	No
	Goal 5: Insight into condition assessed			
	Aware of diagnosis a) Patient	❑	❑	❑
	b) Family/Other		❑	❑
	Recognition of dying c) Patient	❑	❑	❑
	d) Family/Other		❑	❑

RELIGIOUS/ SPIRITUAL SUPPORT	**Goal 6: Religious/spiritual needs assessed with patient/carer** Yes ❑ No ❑ Formal religion identified: .... In-house support Tel/Bleep No: .... Name .... External support Tel/Bleep No: .... Name .... Special needs now, at time of & after death identified:- (please state) ....
COMMUNICATION WITH FAMILY/OTHER	**Goal 7: Identify how family/other are to be informed of patient's impending death** Yes ❑ No ❑ At any time ❑ Not at night-time ❑ Stay overnight at Hospital ❑ Primary Contact Name .... Relationship to patient .... Tel no: .... Secondary contact .... Tel no: ....
	Goal 8: Family/other given hospital information on:- Yes ❑ No ❑ Concession car parking; Hillsborough accommodation; Dining Room facilities; Payphones; Washrooms & toilet facilities on the ward. Any other relevant information
COMMUNICATION WITH PRIMARY HEALTH CARE TEAM	**Goal 9: G.P. Practice is aware of patient's condition** Yes ❑ No ❑ G.P. Practice to be contacted if unaware patient is dying
SUMMARY	**Goal 10: Plan of care explained & discussed with:-** a) Patient ❑ b) Family ❑ c) Other ❑ d) No ❑
	Goal 11: Family/other express understanding of plan care Yes ❑ No ❑ N/A ❑

If you have charted "No" against any goal so far, please complete variance sheet on the back page before signing below

Signature Health Care Professional　　　　　　**Title**　　　　　**Date**

INTEGRATED CARE PATHWAY FOR THE TERMINAL/DYING PHASE

NAME: .... UNIT NO: .... DATE: ....

Codes (Please enter in columns) A.. Achieved   V.. Variance

SECTION 2	PATIENT PROBLEM/FOCUS	08:00	12:00	16:00	20:00	24:00	04:00
ASSESSMENT PAIN/COMFORT MEASURES							
Pain **Goal: Patient is pain free** ● Verbalised by patient if conscious ● Pain free on movement ● Appears peaceful ● Move only for comfort							
Agitation **Goal: Patient is not agitated** ● Patient does not display signs of delirium, terminal anguish, restlessness (thrashing, plucking, twitching) ● Exclude retention of urine as cause							
Respiratory Tract Secretions **Goal: Patients breathing is not made difficult by excessive secretions**							
Nausea & Vomiting **Goal: Patient does not feel nauseous or vomits** ● Patient verbalises if conscious							
Other symptoms (e.g. dyspnoea) a)							
TREATMENT/PROCEDURES							
Mouth Care **Goal: Mouth is moist and clean.** ● See mouth care policy ● Mouth care to be given at least 4 hourly							
Micturition Difficulties **Goal: Patient is comfortable** ● Urinary catheter if in retention ● Urinary catheter or pads, if general weakness creates incontinence							
MEDICATION (If not appropriate record as N/A)							
Goal: All medication is given safely & accurately. ● If syringe driver in progress check at least 4 hourly ● If medication not required please record as N/A							
Nurse Signature		Early		Late		Night	
Repeat this page 24 hrly. Spare copies on Ward							

INTEGRATED CARE PATHWAY FOR THE TERMINAL/DYING PHASE

NAME: .... UNIT NO: .... DATE: ....

Complete **12 hourly**		08:00	20:00
MOBILITY/PRESSURE AREA CARE	**Goal: Patient is comfortable and in a safe environment** Patient is moved for comfort only with pressure relieving aids as appropriate e.g. special mattress		
BOWEL CARE	**Goal: Patient is not agitated or distressed due to constipation or diarrhoea**		
PSYCHOLOGICAL/ INSIGHT SUPPORT	**Patient** **Goal: Patient becomes aware of the situation as appropriate** ● Patient is informed of procedures ● Touch, verbal communication is continued		
	Family/Other **Goal: Family/Other are prepared for the patient's imminent death with the aim of achieving peace of mind and acceptance** ● Check understanding ● Recognition of patient dying ● Inform of measures taken to maintain patient's comfort ● Explain possibility of physical symptoms e.g. fatigue ● Psychological symptoms such as anxiety/depression ● Social issues such as financial implications		
RELIGIOUS/SPIRITUAL SUPPORT	**Goal: Appropriate religious/spiritual support has been given**		
CARE OF THE FAMILY/OTHERS	**Goal: The needs of those attending the patient are accommodated**		

IF YOU HAVE CHARTERED 'V' AGAINST ANY GOAL SO FAR, PLEASE COMPLETE VARIANCE SHEET AT THE BACK OF THE PATHWAY BEFORE SIGNING BELOW
Repeat this page each 24 hours. Spare sheets on Ward

Nurse Signature   Early .... Late .... Night ....

MULTIDISCIPLINARY PROGRESS NOTES

INTEGRATED CARE PATHWAY FOR THE TERMINAL/DYING PHASE

NAME: .... UNIT NO: .... DATE: ....

Codes (Please enter in columns) A.. Achieved   V.. Variance

SECTION 2	PATIENT PROBLEM/FOCUS	08:00	12:00	16:00	20:00	24:00	04:00
ASSESSMENT PAIN/COMFORT MEASURES							
Pain **Goal: Patient is pain free** • Verbalised by patient if conscious • Pain free on movement • Appears peaceful • Move only for comfort							
Agitation **Goal: Patient is not agitated** • Patient does not display signs of delirium, terminal anguish, restlessness (thrashing, plucking, twitching) • Exclude retention of urine as cause							
Respiratory Tract Secretions **Goal: Patients breathing is not made difficult by excessive secretions**							
Nausea & Vomiting **Goal: Patient does not feel nauseous or vomits** • Patient verbalises if conscious							
Other symptoms (e.g. dyspnoea) a)							
TREATMENT/PROCEDURES							
Mouth Care **Goal: Mouth is moist and clean.** • See mouth care policy • Mouth care to be given at least 4 hourly							
Micturition Difficulties **Goal: Patient is comfortable** • Urinary catheter if in retention • Urinary catheter or pads, if general weakness creates incontinence							
MEDICATION (If not appropriate record as N/A)							
Goal: All medication is given safely & accurately. • If syringe driver in progress check at least 4 hourly • If medication not required please record as N/A							
Nurse Signature **Repeat this page 24 hrly. Spare copies on Ward**		Early		Late		Night	

INTEGRATED CARE PATHWAY FOR THE TERMINAL/DYING PHASE

NAME: .... UNIT NO: .... DATE: ....

Complete **12 hourly**		08:00	20:00
MOBILITY/PRESSURE AREA CARE	**Goal: Patient is comfortable and in a safe environment** Patient is moved for comfort only with pressure relieving aids as appropriate e.g. special mattress		
BOWEL CARE	**Goal: Patient is not agitated or distressed due to constipation or diarrhoea**		
PSYCHOLOGICAL/ INSIGHT SUPPORT	**Patient** **Goal: Patient becomes aware of the situation as appropriate** • Patient is informed of procedures • Touch, verbal communication is continued		
	Family/Other **Goal: Family/Other are prepared for the patient's imminent death with the aim of achieving peace of mind and acceptance** • Check understanding • Recognition of patient dying • Inform of measures taken to maintain patient's comfort • Explain possibility of physical symptoms e.g. fatigue • Psychological symptoms such as anxiety/depression • Social issues such as financial implications		
RELIGIOUS/SPIRITUAL SUPPORT	**Goal: Appropriate religious/spiritual support has been given**		
CARE OF THE FAMILY/OTHERS	**Goal: The needs of those attending the patient are accommodated**		

IF YOU HAVE CHARTERED 'V' AGAINST ANY GOAL SO FAR, PLEASE COMPLETE VARIANCE SHEET AT THE BACK OF THE PATHWAY BEFORE SIGNING BELOW
Repeat this page each 24 hours. Spare sheets on Ward

Nurse Signature   Early ....   Late ....   Night ....

MULTIDISCIPLINARY PROGRESS NOTES

INTEGRATED CARE PATHWAY FOR THE TERMINAL/DYING PHASE

NAME: .... UNIT NO: .... DATE: ....

VERIFICATION OF DEATH

Date of Death .... Time of Death ....

Persons Present ....

Notes ....

....

Signature .... Time Verified ....

CARE AFTER DEATH	
Goal 12: GP Practice contacted re patient's death Date: _/_/_	Yes ❑ No ❑
Goal 13: Procedures for laying out followed according to hospital policy ● **Input patients death on hospital computer**	Yes ● No ❑
Goal 14: Procedure following death discussed or carried out N/A ❑ **(If yes please indicate)** Patient had infectious disease ❑ Patient has religious needs ❑ Post mortem discussed ❑	Yes ❑ No ❑
Goal 15: Family/other given information on hospital procedures ● Hospital information booklet given to Family/Other about necessary legal tasks ● Relatives/other informed to ring General Office at 10am on next working day to make an appointment to collect death certificate	Yes ❑ No ❑
Goal 16: Hospital policy followed for patient's valuabes & belongings **OUT OF OFFICE HOURS** ● Belongings listed and put in A&E Clothing Store ● Vluables listed and put in A&E night safe **IN OFFICE HOURS** ● Belongings & valuables listed & taken to General Office	Yes ❑ No ❑
Goal 17: Necessary documentation & advice is given to the **appropriate person** ● General office booklet given	Yes ❑ No ❑
Goal 18: Bereavement leaflet given ● 'What to do after death' booklet given (DHSS) if applicable ● Grieving leaflet given	Yes ❑ No ❑
IF YOU HAVE CHARTED "NO" AGAINST ANY GOAL SO FAR, PLEASE COMPLETE VARIANCE SHEET AT THE BACK OF THE PATHWAY BEFORE SIGNING BELOW Nurse Signature .... Date	
***** **HAVE YOU COMPLETED THE LAST 4 & 12 HOURLY OBSERVATION**	
PLEASE CONTACT THE PALLIATIVE CARE TEAM TO INFORM THEM THAT THIS PATIENT WAS ON A PATHWAY. EXT 2274	

INTEGRATED CARE PATHWAY FOR THE TERMINAL/DYING PHASE

NAME: .... UNIT NO: .... DATE: ....

VARIANCE ANALYSIS FOR TERMINAL/DYING PHASE

HOSPITAL

CONSULTANT: ....
DATE OF ADMISSION: ....
DATE OF DEATH: ....
WARD: ....

DATE	WHAT VARIANCE OCCURRED?	WHY DID VARIANCE OCCUR?	ACTION TAKEN	INITIALS	TITLE

Appendix 2

LCP—Hospice

NAME: .... UNIT NO: ....

HOSPICE

THE LIVERPOOL INTEGRATED CARE PATHWAY FOR THE TERMINAL/DYING PHASE

A Care Pathway is intended as a guide to treatment and an aid to documenting patient progress. Of course, practitioners are free to exercise their own professional judgement, however any alteration to the practice identified within this ICP must be noted as a variance on the sheet at the back of the pathway.

*Reference: Changing Gear – Guidelines for Managing the Last Days of Life in Adults. National Council for Hospice and Specialist Palliative Care Services. Northamptonshire: Land & Unwin (Data Sciences) Ltd, 1997

CONSULTANT: **NAMED NURSE:**   **WARD:**

INSTRUCTIONS FOR USE

1. All goals are in **heavy** typeface. Interventions, which act as prompts to support the goals, are in normal type.

2. If a goal is not achieved (i.e. variance) then chart on the variance section on the back page.

3. At the end of the patient episode review ICP, any goals that are not achieved should be charted as a variance in the variance section at the end of each 24 hour assessment page.

4. Please record all other multi-disciplinary information In the multi-disciplinary progress notes section.

ALL PERSONNEL COMPLETING THE CARE PATHWAY PLEASE SIGN BELOW

Name (Print)	Full Signature	Initials	Professional Title	Date

CRITERIA FOR ICP – DO NOT PUT ON THE PATHWAY UNLESS

The Multidisciplinary team have agreed the patient is dying and two of the following apply:-

The patient is bedbound   ❏   Semi-Comatose   ❏

Only able to take sips of fluids   ❏   No longer able to take tablets   ❏

INTEGRATED CARE PATHWAY FOR THE TERMINAL/DYING PHASE

NAME: .... UNIT NO: .... DATE: ....

SECTION 1	PATIENT ASSESSMENT	
COMFORT MEASURES	(If 'No' chart as variance on the back page) **Goal 1: Current medication assessed and non essentials discontinued** Appropriate oral drugs converted to subcutaneous route and syringe driver commenced if appropriate Inappropriate medication discontinued	Yes ❑ No ❑

	Goal 2: PRN subcutaneous medication written up as per regional
	           Standards & Guidelines
	    Agitation Pain Analgesia Sedative
	    Respiratory Tract Secretions Nausea & Vomiting Anti–emetic Anticholinergic
		Yes ❑ No ❑

	Goal 3: Discontinue inappropriate interventions
	    Blood Test
	    Antibiotics
	    I.V.'s (fluids/medications)
		Yes ❑ No ❑

	Doctor's signature .... Date	
PSYCHOLOGICAL/ INSIGHT	**Goal 4: Ability to communicate in English assessed as adequate**	Yes ❑ No ❑

	Goal 5: Insight into condition assessed: Comatosed Yes No
	         Aware of diagnosis: a) Patient ❑ ❑ ❑
	                                        b) Family/Other ❑ ❑
	
	         Recognition of dying: c) Patient ❑ ❑ ❑
	                                        d) Family/Other ❑ ❑	

RELIGIOUS/ SPIRITUAL SUPPORT	**Goal 6: Religious/spiritual needs assessed with patient/carer** Formal religion identified: .... No formal religion ❑ In-house support Tel/Bleep No: .... Name .... External support Tel/Bleep No: .... Name .... Special needs now, at time of & after death identified:- (please state)	Yes ❑ No ❑
COMMUNICATION WITH FAMILY/OTHER	**Goal 7: Identify how family/other are to be informed of patient's** **impending death** At any time ❑ Not at night-time ❑ Stay overnight at Hospice ❑ Primary Contact Name .... Relationship to patient .... Tel no: .... Secondary contact .... Tel no:	Yes ❑ No ❑
	Goal 8: Family/other given Hospice facilities leaflet:	Yes ❑ No ❑
COMMUNICATION WITH PRIMARY HEALTH CARE TEAM	**Goal 9: G.P. Practice is aware of patient's condition** G.P. Practice to be contacted if unaware patient is dying	Yes ❑ No ❑
SUMMARY	**Goal 10: Plan of care explained & discussed with:-** a) Patient ❑ b) Family ❑ c) Other ❑ d) No ❑	
	Goal 11: Family/other express understanding **of plan care** Not Applicable ❑ Yes ❑ No ❑	
If you have charted "No" against any goal so far, please complete variance sheet on the back page before signing below		
Signature Health Care Professional Title Date		

INTEGRATED CARE PATHWAY FOR THE TERMINAL/DYING PHASE

NAME: .... UNIT NO: .... DATE: ....

Codes (Please enter in columns) A.. Achieved   V.. Variance

SECTION 2	PATIENT PROBLEM/FOCUS	08:00	12:00	16:00	20:00	24:00	04:00
ASSESSMENT PAIN/COMFORT MEASURES							
Pain **Goal: Patient is pain free** ● Verbalised by patient if conscious ● Pain free on movement ● Appears peaceful ● Move only for comfort							
Agitation **Goal: Patient is not agitated** ● Patient does not display signs of delirium, terminal anguish, restlessness (thrashing, plucking, twitching) ● Exclude retention of urine as cause							
Respiratory Tract Secretions **Goal: Patients breathing is not made difficult by excessive secretions**							
Nausea & Vomiting **Goal: Patient does not feel nauseous or vomits** ● Patient verbalises if conscious							
Other symptoms (e.g. dyspnoea) a)							
TREATMENT/PROCEDURES							
Mouth Care **Goal: Mouth is moist and clean.** ● Mouth care to be given at least 4 hourly							
Micturition Difficulties **Goal: Patient is comfortable** ● Urinary catheter if in retention ● Urinary catheter or pads, if general weakness creates incontinence							
MEDICATION (If not appropriate record as N/A)							
Goal: All medication is given safely & accurately. ● All appropriate syringe driver medications given as prescribed and syringe driver checked at least 4 hourly ● Other medication is delivered safely and accurately as prescribed. (If not appropriate please record as N/A)							
Please initial each shift: **Repeat this page 24 hrly. Spare copies on Ward**	Early		Late		Night		

INTEGRATED CARE PATHWAY FOR THE TERMINAL/DYING PHASE

NAME: .... UNIT NO: .... DATE: ....

Complete **12 hourly**		08:00	20:00
MOBILITY/PRESSURE AREA CARE	**Goal: Patient is comfortable and in a safe environment** Patient is moved for comfort only with pressure relieving aids as appropriate e.g. special mattress		
BOWEL CARE	**Goal: Patient is not agitated or distressed due to constipation or diarrhoea**		
PSYCHOLOGICAL/ INSIGHT SUPPORT	**Patient** **Goal: Patient becomes aware of the situation as appropriate** ● Patient is informed of procedures ● Touch, verbal communication is continued		
	Family/Other **Goal: Family/Other are prepared for the patient's imminent death with the aim of achieving peace of mind and acceptance** ● Check understanding ● Recognition of patient dying ● Inform of measures taken to maintain patient's comfort		
RELIGIOUS/SPIRITUAL SUPPORT	**Goal: Appropriate religious/spiritual support has been given**		
CARE OF THE FAMILY/OTHERS	**Goal: The needs of those attending the patient are accommodated**		

IF YOU HAVE CHARTERED 'V' AGAINST ANY GOAL SO FAR, PLEASE COMPLETE VARIANCE SHEET AT THE BACK OF THE PATHWAY BEFORE SIGNING BELOW
Repeat this page each 24 hours. Spare sheets on Ward

Please inital each shift: Early .... Late .... Night ....

MULTIDISCIPLINARY PROGRESS NOTES

INTEGRATED CARE PATHWAY FOR THE TERMINAL/DYING PHASE

NAME: .... UNIT NO: .... DATE: ....

Codes (Please enter in columns) A.. Achieved   V.. Variance

SECTION 2	PATIENT PROBLEM/FOCUS	08:00	12:00	16:00	20:00	24:00	04:00
ASSESSMENT PAIN/COMFORT MEASURES							
Pain **Goal: Patient is pain free** ● Verbalised by patient if conscious ● Pain free on movement ● Appears peaceful ● Move only for comfort							
Agitation **Goal: Patient is not agitated** ● Patient does not display signs of delirium, terminal anguish, restlessness (thrashing, plucking, twitching) ● Exclude retention of urine as cause							
Respiratory Tract Secretions **Goal: Patients breathing is not made difficult by** excessive secretions							
Nausea & Vomiting **Goal: Patient does not feel nauseous or vomits** ● Patient verbalises if conscious							
Other symptoms (e.g. dyspnoea) a)							
TREATMENT/PROCEDURES							
Mouth Care **Goal: Mouth is moist and clean.** ● Mouth care to be given at least 4 hourly							
Micturition Difficulties **Goal: Patient is comfortable** ● Urinary catheter if in retention ● Urinary catheter or pads, if general weakness creates incontinence							
MEDICATION (If not appropriate record as N/A)							
Goal: All medication is given safely & accurately. ● All appropriate syringe driver medications given as prescribed and syringe driver checked at least 4 hourly ● Other medication is delivered safely and accurately as prescribed. (If not appropriate please record as N/A)							
Please initial each shift: **Repeat this page 24 hrly. Spare copies on Ward**	Early		Late		Night		

INTEGRATED CARE PATHWAY FOR THE TERMINAL/DYING PHASE

NAME: .... UNIT NO: .... DATE: ....

Complete **12 hourly**		08:00	20:00
MOBILITY/PRESSURE AREA CARE	**Goal: Patient is comfortable and in a safe environment** Patient is moved for comfort only with pressure relieving aids as appropriate e.g. special mattress		
BOWEL CARE	**Goal: Patient is not agitated or distressed due to constipation or diarrhoea**		
PSYCHOLOGICAL/ INSIGHT SUPPORT	**Patient** **Goal: Patient becomes aware of the situation as appropriate** ● Patient is informed of procedures ● Touch, verbal communication is continued		
	Family/Other **Goal: Family/Other are prepared for the patient's imminent death with the aim of achieving peace of mind and acceptance** ● Check understanding ● Recognition of patient dying ● Inform of measures taken to maintain patient's comfort		
RELIGIOUS/SPIRITUAL SUPPORT	**Goal: Appropriate religious/spiritual support has been given**		
CARE OF THE FAMILY/OTHERS	**Goal: The needs of those attending the patient are accommodated**		

IF YOU HAVE CHARTERED 'V' AGAINST ANY GOAL SO FAR, PLEASE COMPLETE VARIANCE SHEET AT THE BACK OF THE PATHWAY BEFORE SIGNING BELOW
Repeat this page each 24 hours.   Spare sheets on Ward

Please inital each shift: Early ....   Late ....   Night ....

MULTIDISCIPLINARY PROGRESS NOTES

INTEGRATED CARE PATHWAY FOR THE TERMINAL/DYING PHASE

NAME: .... UNIT NO: .... DATE: ....

VERIFICATION OF DEATH

Date of Death .... Time of Death ....

Persons Present ....

Nurse Signature ....

Cause of Death ....

Doctors Signature .... Time Verified ....

CARE AFTER DEATH	**Goal 12: GP Practice contacted re patient's death** ● G.P. letter completed	Yes ☐ No ☐
	Goal 13: Procedures for laying out followed according to Hospital policy ● Opportunities for viewing explained	Yes ☐ No ☐
	Goal 14: Procedure following death discussed or carried out N/A ☐ **(If yes please indicate)** Patient had infectious disease ☐ Patient has religious needs ☐ Post mortem discussed ☐	Yes ☐ No ☐
	Goal 15: Family/other given information on hospital procedures ● Advised to telephone prior to returning to Hospice ● Patients death input on Pal-care computer	Yes ☐ No ☐
	Goal 16: Belongings and valuables are signed for by identified person ● Property packed for collection ● Valuables listed and stored safely	Yes ☐ No ☐
	Goal 17: Necessary documentation & advice is given to the appropriate person ● Death Certificate signed ● Need for cremation certificate explained (2 doctors to sign) ● Coroner notified when necessary ● Aid with funeral expenses (assisted as identified) ● Confirm understanding of need to register death	Yes ☐ No ☐
	Goal 18: Bereavement referral form completed ● 'What to do after death' booklet given (DHSS) if applicable ● Bereavement and support leaflet given ● Hospice leaflet given (registering a death)	Yes ☐ No ☐
	IF YOU HAVE CHARTED "NO" AGAINST ANY GOAL SO FAR, PLEASE COMPLETE VARIANCE SHEET AT THE BACK OF THE PATHWAY BEFORE SIGNING BELOW **Nurse Signature** .... **Date** .... *** HAVE YOU COMPLETED THE LAST 4 & 12 HOURLY OBSERVATION** Yes ☐ No ☐	

INTEGRATED CARE PATHWAY FOR THE TERMINAL/DYING PHASE

NAME: .... DOB: .... DATE: ....

VARIANCE ANALYSIS FOR TERMINAL/DYING PHASE

HOSPICE

G.P.: ....
DATE OF DEATH: ....

DATE	WHAT VARIANCE OCCURRED?	WHY DID VARIANCE OCCUR?	ACTION TAKEN	INITIALS	TITLE

Appendix 3

LCP—Community

NAME: .... DOB: ....

GENERIC COMMUNITY PATHWAY

THE LIVERPOOL INTEGRATED CARE PATHWAY FOR THE TERMINAL/DYING PHASE

A Care Pathway is intended as a guide to treatment and an aid to documenting patient progress. Of course, practitioners are free to exercise their own professional judgement, however any alteration to the practice identified within this ICP must be noted as a variance on the sheet at the back of the pathway.

> *Reference: Changing Gear – Guidelines for Managing the Last Days of Life in Adults. National Council for Hospice and Specialist Palliative Care Services. Northamptonshire: Land & Unwin (Data Sciences) Ltd, 1997

G.P: **NAMED NURSE:**

INSTRUCTIONS FOR USE   **PRIMARY CARE TRUST:**

1.   All goals are in **heavy** typeface. Interventions, which act as prompts to support the goals, are in normal type.

2.   If a goal is not achieved (i.e. variance) then chart on the variance section on the back page.

3.   The Palliative Care guidelines are printed on the pages at the end of the pathway. Please make reference as necessary.

4.   If you have any problems regarding the Pathway contact the Macmillan Nurse.

ALL PERSONNEL COMPLETING THE CARE PATHWAY PLEASE SIGN BELOW

Name (Print)	Full Signature	Initials	Professional Title	Date

CRITERIA FOR ICP – DO NOT PUT ON THE PATHWAY UNLESS

The Multiprofessional team have agreed the patient is dying and two of the following apply:-

The patient is bedbound   ❏   Semi-Comatose   ❏

Only able to take sips of fluids   ❏   No longer able to take tablets   ❏

LIVERPOOL INTEGRATED CARE PATHWAY FOR THE DYING PHASE

INTEGRATED CARE PATHWAY FOR THE TERMINAL/DYING PHASE

NAME: .... DOB: .... DATE: ....

SECTION 1	PATIENT ASSESSMENT					

	PRIMARY			SECONDARY		
DIAGNOSIS	Ethnicity					

PHYSICAL CONDITION	Unable to swallow	Yes ❑	No ❑	Aware	Yes ❑	No ❑
	Nausea	Yes ❑	No ❑	Conscious	Yes ❑	No ❑
	Vomiting	Yes ❑	No ❑	UTI Problems	Yes ❑	No ❑
	Constipated	Yes ❑	No ❑	Catheterised	Yes ❑	No ❑
	Confused	Yes ❑	No ❑	Respiratory Tract Secretions	Yes ❑	No ❑
	Agitation	Yes ❑	No ❑	Dyspnoea	Yes ❑	No ❑
	Restless	Yes ❑	No ❑	Pain	Yes ❑	No ❑
	Distressed	Yes ❑	No ❑	Other	Yes ❑	No ❑

COMFORT MEASURES	**Goal 1: Current medication assessed and non essentials discontinued** Yes ❑ No ❑
	Appropriate oral drugs converted to subcutaneous route and syringe driver commenced if appropriate
	Inappropriate medication discontinued

	Goal 2: PRN subcutaneous medication written up for list below as per Protocol Yes ❑ No ❑
	Pain Analgesia
	Nausea & Vomiting Anti-emetic
	Agitation Sedative
	Respiratory Tract Secretions Anticholinergic

	Goal 3: Discontinue inappropriate interventions Yes ❑ No ❑
	Blood Test
	Antibiotics

	Doctor's signature ....….......... Date ....

	Goal 3a: Decisions to discontinue inappropriate nursing interventions taken Yes ❑ No ❑
	Routine Turning Regime (turn for comfort only)
	Taking Vital signs

	Goal 3b: Syringe driver set up within 4 hours of identified need Yes ❑ No ❑ N/A ❑
	Nurse signature .... Date .... Time ....

If you have charted "No" against any goal so far, please complete variance sheet on the back page

INTEGRATED CARE PATHWAY FOR THE TERMINAL/DYING PHASE

NAME: .... DOB: .... DATE: ....

SECTION 1	Patient assessment Contd/			
PSYCHOLOGICAL/ INSIGHT	**Goal 4: Ability to communicate in English assessed as adequate**		Yes ❑	No ❑
	Goal 5: Insight into condition assessed	Comatosed	Yes	No
	Aware of diagnosis a) Patient	❑	❑	❑
	b) Family/Other		❑	❑
	Recognition of dying c) Patient	❑	❑	❑
	d) Family/Other		❑	❑
RELIGIOUS/ SPIRITUAL SUPPORT	**Goal 6: Religious/spiritual needs assessed with patient/carer** Yes ❑ No ❑ Formal religion identified: --- Special needs now, at time of & after death identified:- (please state) -- -- --			
COMMUNICATION WITH FAMILY/OTHER	**Goal 7: Family/other given hospital information on:-** Not to call emergency ambulance Not to attempt to resuscitate Contact numbers for 24 hour cover		Yes ❑	No ❑
COMMUNICATION WITH PRIMARY HEALTH CARE TEAM	**Goal 8: G.P. Practice is aware of patient's condition** G.P. Practice to be contacted if unaware patient is dying		Yes ❑	No ❑
SUMMARY	**Goal 9: Plan of care explained & discussed with:-** a) Patient ❑ b) Family ❑ c) Other ❑ d) No ❑			
	Goal 10: Family/other express understanding of plan care Yes ❑ No ❑ N/A ❑ Family/carer involvement in physical care			
If you have charted "No" against any goal so far, please complete variance sheet on the back page before signing below				
Signature Health Care Professional Title Date				

INTEGRATED CARE PATHWAY FOR THE TERMINAL/DYING PHASE

NAME: .... DOB: ....

Codes (Please enter in columns) A= Achieved V= Variance							
SECTION 2	**PATIENT PROBLEM/FOCUS** **Record time of vist**	Date	Date	Date	Date	Date	Date
ASSESSMENT **PAIN/COMFORT MEASURES**		Time	Time	Time	Time	Time	Time
Pain **Goal: Patient is pain free** ● Verbalised by patient if conscious ● Pain free on movement ● Appears peaceful ● Move only for comfort							
Agitation **Goal: Patient is not agitated** ● Patient does not display signs of delirium, terminal anguish, restlessness (thrashing, plucking, twitching) ● Exclude retention of urine as cause							
Respiratory Tract Secretions **Goal: Patients breathing is not made difficult by excessive secretions**							
Nausea & Vomiting **Goal: Patient does not feel nauseous or vomits** ● Patient verbalises if conscious							
Other symptoms (e.g. dyspnoea) a)							
TREATMENT/PROCEDURES							
Mouth Care **Goal: Mouth is moist and clean.** ● See mouth care policy ● Mouth care to be given at least 4 hourly							
Micturition Difficulties **Goal: Patient is comfortable** ● Urinary catheter if in retention ● Urinary catheter or pads, if general weakness creates incontinence							
MEDICATION (If not appropriate record as N/A)							
Goal: All medication is given safely & accurately. ● If syringe driver in progress check each visit ● If medication not required please record as N/A							
Nurse Signature							
If you have charted "V" against any goal so far, please complete variance sheet on the back page							

INTEGRATED CARE PATHWAY FOR THE TERMINAL/DYING PHASE

NAME: .... DOB: ....

		Date	Date	Date	Date	Date	Date
		Time	Time	Time	Time	Time	Time
MOBILITY/PRESSURE AREA CARE	Goal: Patient is comfortable and in a safe environment Patient is moved for comfort only with pressure relieving aids as appropriate e.g. special mattress						
BOWEL CARE	Goal: Patient is not agitated or distressed due to constipation or diarrhoea						
PSYCHOLOGICAL/ INSIGHT SUPPORT	Patient Goal: Patient becomes aware of the situation as appropriate ● Patient is informed of procedures ● Touch, verbal communication is continued						
	Family/Other Goal: Family/Other are prepared For the patient's imminent Death with the aim of achieving peace of mind and acceptance ● Check understanding ● Recognition of patient dying ● Inform of measures taken to maintain patient's comfort ● Explain possibility of physical symptoms e.g. fatigue ● Psychological symptoms such as anxiety/depression ● Social issues such as financial implications						
RELIGIOUS/SPIRITUAL SUPPORT	Goal: Appropriate religious/ spiritual support has been given						
CARE OF THE FAMILY/OTHERS	Goal: The needs of those attending the patient are accommodated						
Nurse Signature							

If you have charted "V" against any goal so far, please complete variance sheet on the back page

INTEGRATED CARE PATHWAY FOR THE TERMINAL/DYING PHASE

NAME: .... DOB: ....

Codes (Please enter in columns) A= Achieved V= Variance						
SECTION 2	**PATIENT PROBLEM/FOCUS** **Record time of vist**	Date	Date	Date	Date	Date	Date
ASSESSMENT **PAIN/COMFORT MEASURES**		Time	Time	Time	Time	Time	Time
Pain **Goal: Patient is pain free** ● Verbalised by patient if conscious ● Pain free on movement ● Appears peaceful ● Move only for comfort							
Agitation **Goal: Patient is not agitated** ● Patient does not display signs of delirium, terminal anguish, restlessness (thrashing, plucking, twitching) ● Exclude retention of urine as cause							
Respiratory Tract Secretions **Goal: Patients breathing is not made difficult by excessive secretions**							
Nausea & Vomiting **Goal: Patient does not feel nauseous or vomits** ● Patient verbalises if conscious							
Other symptoms (e.g. dyspnoea) a)							
TREATMENT/PROCEDURES							
Mouth Care **Goal: Mouth is moist and clean.** ● See mouth care policy ● Mouth care to be given at least 4 hourly							
Micturition Difficulties **Goal: Patient is comfortable** ● Urinary catheter if in retention ● Urinary catheter or pads, if general weakness creates incontinence							
MEDICATION (If not appropriate record as N/A)							
Goal: All medication is given safely & accurately. ● If syringe driver in progress check each visit ● If medication not required please record as N/A							
Nurse Signature							
If you have charted "V" against any goal so far, please complete variance sheet on the back page							

INTEGRATED CARE PATHWAY FOR THE TERMINAL/DYING PHASE

NAME: .... DOB: ....

		Date Time	Date Time	Date Time	Date Time	Date Time	Date Time
MOBILITY/PRESSURE AREA CARE	Goal: Patient is comfortable and in a safe environment Patient is moved for comfort only with pressure relieving aids as appropriate e.g. special mattress						
BOWEL CARE	Goal: Patient is not agitated or distressed due to constipation or diarrhoea						
PSYCHOLOGICAL/ INSIGHT SUPPORT	Patient Goal: Patient becomes aware of the situation as appropriate ● Patient is informed of procedures ● Touch, verbal communication is continued						
	Family/Other Goal: Family/Other are prepared For the patient's imminent Death with the aim of achieving peace of mind and acceptance ● Check understanding ● Recognition of patient dying ● Inform of measures taken to maintain patient's comfort ● Explain possibility of physical symptoms e.g. fatigue ● Psychological symptoms such as anxiety/depression ● Social issues such as financial implications						
RELIGIOUS/SPIRITUAL SUPPORT	Goal: Appropriate religious/ spiritual support has been given						
CARE OF THE FAMILY/OTHERS	Goal: The needs of those attending the patient are accommodated						
Nurse Signature							

If you have charted "V" against any goal so far, please complete variance sheet on the back page

INTEGRATED CARE PATHWAY FOR THE TERMINAL/DYING PHASE

NAME: .... DOB: .... DATE:..............................

TIME/DATE	MULTIDISCIPLINARY PROGRESS NOTES	SIGNATURE
	COMMENT	

INTEGRATED CARE PATHWAY FOR THE TERMINAL/DYING PHASE

NAME: .... D.O.B: .... DATE: ....

VERIFICATION OF DEATH

Date of Death .... **Time of Death** ....

Persons Present ....

Notes ....

....

Signature .... **Time Verified** ....

CARE AFTER DEATH	Goal 12: GP Practice contacted re patient's death Date: __/__/__	Yes ❐ No ❐
	Goal 13: Procedures for laying out followed	Yes ❐ No ❐
	Goal 14: Procedure following death discussed or carried out N/A ❐ (If yes please indicate) Patient had infectious disease ❐ Patient has religious needs ❐ Post mortem discussed ❐	Yes ❐ No ❐
	Goal 15: Necessary documentation & advice is given to the appropriate person ● Information leaflet on Bereavement/Support Groups given ● Advised to contact registrar to make an appointment ● Contact number for care practitioner involved	Yes ❐ No ❐
	IF YOU HAVE CHARTED "NO" AGAINST ANY GOAL SO FAR, PLEASE COMPLETE VARIANCE SHEET AT THE BACK OF THE PATHWAY BEFORE SIGNING BELOW **Nurse Signature** .... **Date**	

INTEGRATED CARE PATHWAY FOR THE TERMINAL/DYING PHASE

NAME: .... DOB: .... DATE: ....

VARIANCE ANALYSIS FOR TERMINAL/DYING PHASE

COMMUNITY ICP

G.P: ....

DATE OF DEATH: ....

DATE	WHAT VARIANCE OCCURRED?	WHY DID VARIANCE OCCUR?	ACTION TAKEN	INITIALS	TITLE

INTEGRATED CARE PATHWAY FOR THE TERMINAL/DYING PHASE

NAME: .... DOB: .... DATE: ....

VARIANCE ANALYSIS FOR TERMINAL/DYING PHASE

COMMUNITY ICP

G.P: ....
DATE OF DEATH: ....

DATE	WHAT VARIANCE OCCURRED?	WHY DID VARIANCE OCCUR?	ACTION TAKEN	INITIALS	TITLE

LCP—Nursing home

NAME: .... DOB: ....

NURSING HOME

THE LIVERPOOL INTEGRATED CARE PATHWAY FOR THE TERMINAL/DYING PHASE
A Care Pathway is intended as a guide to treatment and an aid to documenting patient progress. Of course, practitioners are free to exercise their own professional judgement, however any alteration to the practice identified within this ICP must be noted as a variance on the sheet at the back of the pathway.

*Reference: Changing Gear – Guidelines for Managing the Last Days of Life in Adults. National Council for Hospice and Specialist Palliative Care Services. Northamptonshire: Land & Unwin (Data Sciences) Ltd, 1997

G.P: **NAMED NURSE:**   **ROOM NO:**

<u>**INSTRUCTIONS FOR USE**</u>

1. All goals are in **heavy** typeface. Interventions, which act as prompts to support the goals, are in normal type.

2. If a goal is not achieved (i.e. variance) then chart on the variance section on the back page.

3. At the end of the patient episode review the ICP, any goals that are not achieved should be charted as a variance on the coloured sheet at the back of the pathway

4. Please record all other multi-disciplinary information in the multi-disciplinary notes section.

ALL PERSONNEL COMPLETING THE CARE PATHWAY PLEASE SIGN BELOW

Name (Print)	Full Signature	Initials	Professional Title	Date

CRITERIA FOR ICP – DO NOT PUT ON THE PATHWAY UNLESS

The Multiprofessional team have agreed the patient is dying and two of the following apply:-

The patient is bedbound   ❏   Semi-Comatose   ❏

Only able to take sips of fluids   ❏   No longer able to take tablets   ❏

INTEGRATED CARE PATHWAY FOR THE TERMINAL/DYING PHASE

NAME: .... DOB: .... DATE: ....

SECTION 1	PATIENT ASSESSMENT

DIAGNOSIS	PRIMARY SECONDARY Date of In-patient admission .... Ethnicity ....

COMFORT MEASURES	**Goal 1: Current medication assessed and non essentials discontinued** Yes ❏ No ❏
	        Appropriate oral drugs converted to subcutaneous route and syringe
	        driver commenced if appropriate
	        Inappropriate medication discontinued

	Goal 2: PRN subcutaneous medication written up for list Yes ❏ No ❏
	        below as per Protocol
	        Pain Sedative Analgesia Anticholinergic
	        Nausea & Vomiting Agitation Anti–emetic Respiratory Tract Secretions

	Goal 3: Discontinue inappropriate interventions Yes ❏ No ❏
	        Blood Test
	        Antibiotics
	        I.V.'s (fluids/medications)
	        Not for Cardiopulmonary Resuscitation (Please record below)
	-- 	
	-- 	

	Goal 3a: Decisions to discontinue inappropriate nursing interventions taken Yes ❏ No ❏
	        Routine Turning Regime (turn for comfort only)
	        Taking Vital Signs

	Goal 3b: Syringe Driver set up within 4 hours of Doctors order Yes ❏ No ❏ **Nurse Signature** .... **Date** .... **Time** ....
PSYCHOLOGICAL/ INSIGHT	**Goal 4: Ability to communicate in English assessed as adequate** Yes ❏ No ❏

		Comatosed	Yes	No
	Goal 5: Insight into condition assessed			
	Aware of diagnosis: a) Patient	❏	❏	❏
	b) Family/Other		❏	❏
	Recognition of dying: c) Patient	❏	❏	❏
	d) Family/Other		❏	❏

RELIGIOUS/ SPIRITUAL SUPPORT	**Goal 6: Religious/spiritual needs assessed with patient/carer** Yes ❏ No ❏ Formal religion identified: .... In-house support Tel/Bleep No: .... Name .... External support Tel/Bleep No: .... Name .... Special needs now, at time of & after death identified:- (please state) ....
COMMUNICATION WITH FAMILY/OTHER	**Goal 7: Identify how family/other are to be informed of patient's** Yes ❏ No ❏ **impending death** At any time ❏ Not at night-time ❏ Stay overnight ❏ Primary Contact Name .... Relationship to patient .... Tel no: .... Secondary contact ....Tel no: ....
	Goal 8: Family/other given facilities leaflet Yes ❏ No ❏

COMMUNICATION WITH PRIMARY HEALTH CARE TEAM	Goal 9: G.P. Practice is aware of patient's condition Yes ❑ No ❑ G.P. Practice to be contacted if unaware patient is dying
SUMMARY	Goal 10: Plan of care explained & discussed with:- a) Patient ❑ b) Family ❑ c) Other ❑ d) No ❑
	Goal 11: Family/other express understanding of plan care Not Applicable ❑ Yes ❑ No ❑
	If you have charted "No" against any goal so far, please complete variance sheet on the back page before signing below
	Health Care Professional **Title** **Date**

INTEGRATED CARE PATHWAY FOR THE TERMINAL/DYING PHASE

NAME: .... DOB: .... DATE: ....

Codes (Please enter in columns) A.. Achieved   V.. Variance

SECTION 2	PATIENT PROBLEM/FOCUS	08:00	12:00	16:00	20:00	24:00	04:00
ASSESSMENT PAIN/COMFORT MEASURES							
Pain **Goal: Patient is pain free** ● Verbalised by patient if conscious ● Pain free on movement ● Appears peaceful ● Move only for comfort							
Agitation **Goal: Patient is not agitated** ● Patient does not display signs of delirium, terminal anguish, restlessness (thrashing, plucking, twitching) ● Exclude retention of urine as cause							
Respiratory Tract Secretions **Goal: Patients breathing is not made difficult by excessive secretions**							
Nausea & Vomiting **Goal: Patient does not feel nauseous or vomits** ● Patient verbalises if conscious							
Other symptoms (e.g. dyspnoea) a)							
TREATMENT/PROCEDURES							
Mouth Care **Goal: Mouth is moist and clean.** ● See mouth care policy ● Mouth care to be given at least 4 hourly							
Micturition Difficulties **Goal: Patient is comfortable** ● Urinary catheter if in retention ● Urinary catheter or pads, if general weakness creates incontinence							
MEDICATION (If not appropriate record as N/A)							
Goal: All medication is given safely & accurately. ● If syringe driver in progress check at least 4 hourly ● If medication not required please record as N/A							
Nurse Signature **Repeat this page 24 hrly.**	Early		Late		Night	

INTEGRATED CARE PATHWAY FOR THE TERMINAL/DYING PHASE

NAME: .... DOB: .... DATE: ....

Complete 12 hourly		08:00	20:00
MOBILITY/PRESSURE AREA CARE	Goal: Patient is comfortable and in a safe environment Patient is moved for comfort only with pressure relieving aids as appropriate e.g. special mattress		
BOWEL CARE	Goal: Patient is not agitated or distressed due to constipation or diarrhoea		
PSYCHOLOGICAL/ INSIGHT SUPPORT	Patient Goal: Patient becomes aware of the situation as appropriate ● Patient is informed of procedures ● Touch, verbal communication is continued		
	Family/Other Goal: Family/Other are prepared for the patient's imminent death with the aim of achieving peace of mind and acceptance ● Check understanding ● Recognition of patient dying ● Inform of measures taken to maintain patient's comfort ● Explain possibility of physical symptoms e.g. fatigue ● Psychological symptoms such as anxiety/depression ● Social issues such as financial implications		
RELIGIOUS/SPIRITUAL SUPPORT	Goal: Appropriate religious/spiritual support has been given		
CARE OF THE FAMILY/OTHERS	Goal: The needs of those attending the patient are accommodated		

IF YOU HAVE CHARTERED 'V' AGAINST ANY GOAL SO FAR, PLEASE COMPLETE VARIANCE SHEET AT THE BACK OF THE PATHWAY BEFORE SIGNING BELOW
Repeat this page each 24 hours.

Nurse Signature Early .... Late .... Night ....

MULTIDISCIPLINARY PROGRESS NOTES

INTEGRATED CARE PATHWAY FOR THE TERMINAL/DYING PHASE

NAME: .... DOB: .... DATE: ....

SECTION 2	PATIENT PROBLEM/FOCUS	08:00	12:00	16:00	20:00	24:00	04:00
ASSESSMENT PAIN/COMFORT MEASURES							
Pain **Goal: Patient is pain free** ● Verbalised by patient if conscious ● Pain free on movement ● Appears peaceful ● Move only for comfort							
Agitation **Goal: Patient is not agitated** ● Patient does not display signs of delirium, terminal anguish, restlessness (thrashing, plucking, twitching) ● Exclude retention of urine as cause							
Respiratory Tract Secretions **Goal: Patients breathing is not made difficult by excessive secretions**							
Nausea & Vomiting **Goal: Patient does not feel nauseous or vomits** ● Patient verbalises if conscious							
Other symptoms (e.g. dyspnoea) a)							
TREATMENT/PROCEDURES							
Mouth Care **Goal: Mouth is moist and clean.** ● See mouth care policy ● Mouth care to be given at least 4 hourly							
Micturition Difficulties **Goal: Patient is comfortable** ● Urinary catheter if in retention ● Urinary catheter or pads, if general weakness creates incontinence							
MEDICATION (If not appropriate record as N/A)							
Goal: All medication is given safely & accurately. ● If syringe driver in progress check at least 4 hourly ● If medication not required please record as N/A							
Nurse Signature **Repeat this page 24 hrly.**		Early		Late		Night	

INTEGRATED CARE PATHWAY FOR THE TERMINAL/DYING PHASE

NAME: .... DOB: .... DATE: ....

Complete **12 hourly**		08:00	20:00
MOBILITY/PRESSURE AREA CARE	**Goal: Patient is comfortable and in a safe environment** Patient is moved for comfort only with pressure relieving aids as appropriate e.g. special mattress		
BOWEL CARE	**Goal: Patient is not agitated or distressed due to constipation or diarrhoea**		
PSYCHOLOGICAL/ INSIGHT SUPPORT	**Patient** **Goal: Patient becomes aware of the situation as appropriate** ● Patient is informed of procedures ● Touch, verbal communication is continued		
	Family/Other **Goal: Family/Other are prepared for the patient's Imminent death with the aim of achieving peace of mind and acceptance** ● Check understanding ● Recognition of patient dying ● Inform of measures taken to maintain patient's comfort ● Explain possibility of physical symptoms e.g. fatigue ● Psychological symptoms such as anxiety/depression ● Social issues such as financial implications		
RELIGIOUS/SPIRITUAL SUPPORT	**Goal: Appropriate religious/spiritual support has been given**		
CARE OF THE FAMILY/OTHERS	**Goal: The needs of those attending the patient are accommodated**		
IF YOU HAVE CHARTERED 'V' AGAINST ANY GOAL SO FAR, PLEASE COMPLETE VARIANCE SHEET AT THE BACK OF THE PATHWAY BEFORE SIGNING BELOW **Repeat this page each 24 hours.**			
Nurse Signature Early .... Late .... Night			

MULTIDISCIPLINARY PROGRESS NOTES

INTEGRATED CARE PATHWAY FOR THE TERMINAL/DYING PHASE

NAME: .... DOB: .... DATE: ....

VERIFICATION OF DEATH

Date of Death .... Time of Death ....

Persons Present ....

Notes ....

....

Signature .... Time Verified ....

CARE AFTER DEATH	**Goal 12: GP Practice contacted re patient's death Date: _/_/_** ● G.P letter completed	Yes ☐ No ☐
	Goal 13: Procedures for laying out according to Nursing Home policy ● Mortuary viewing explained	Yes ☐ No ☐
	Goal 14: Procedure following death discussed or carried out N/A ☐ **(If yes please indicate)** Patient had infectious disease ☐ Patient has religious needs ☐ Post mortem discussed ☐	Yes ☐ No ☐
	Goal 15: Family/other given information on procedures ● To contact G.P Surgery to arrange collection of death certificate ● To contact registrars office to arrange a time to register death	Yes ☐ No ☐
	Goal 16: Nursing Hospital policy followed for patient's **valuabes & belongings** ● Belongings to be listed and bagged in patients room ● Valuables listed and put in safe	Yes ☐ No ☐
	Goal 17: Necessary documentation & advice is given to the **appropriate person** ● Pension book returned to DSS ● Notification of death form to be completed and sent to health authority ● Death entered in patients register	Yes ☐ No ☐
	Goal 18: Bereavement leaflet given ● 'What to do after death' booklet given (DHSS) if applicable ● Information leaflet on bereavement and support given	Yes ☐ No ☐
	IF YOU HAVE CHARTED "NO" AGAINST ANY GOAL SO FAR, PLEASE COMPLETE VARIANCE SHEET AT THE BACK OF THE PATHWAY BEFORE SIGNING BELOW **Nurse Signature .... Date ....** **** HAVE YOU COMPLETED THE LAST 4 & 12 HOURLY OBSERVATION***	

INTEGRATED CARE PATHWAY FOR THE TERMINAL/DYING PHASE

NAME: .... DOB: .... DATE: ....

VARIANCE ANALYSIS FOR TERMINAL/DYING PHASE

NURSING HOME

G.P.: ....

DATE OF ADMISSION: ....

DATE OF DEATH: ....

DATE	WHAT VARIANCE OCCURRED?	WHY DID VARIANCE OCCUR?	ACTION TAKEN	INITIALS	TITLE

Appendix 5

Facilities leaflet

The Royal Liverpool and **NHS**
Broadgreen University Hospitals
NHS Trust.

Relative/Carer

Information Leaflet

NHS

REP413.BL.03/98Rev07/00 Review March 2001

Enquiries

If you have any questions or queries please do not hesitate to speak with a member of staff.

Please feel free to contact the ward at any time if you have any concerns.

It is very helpful to the ward team if you ensure that they have your correct name, contact number and address.

It is sometimes easier to cope with this situation if you have someone outside your immediate family to talk to...

The Hospital Palliative Care Team can be contacted by your ward nurse if we can be of help or support at this time.

This leaflet will tell you about the services and facilities available to you whilst you are spending such a great deal of time with your loved one here at the hospital.

Transport

car park facilities

If you are travelling to visit by car, and making repeated journeys to the Hospital then concessional parking facilities may be available. A £3 weekly or £10 monthly parking ticket is available.
Please discuss this further with the ward nurse.

public transport

Merseytravel Hospital Services Timetables can be made available via the main reception desk at the Hospital entrance.

Facilities / Refreshments

shop

The League Of Friends shop is on the first floor concourse and is open Mon-Fri 10.00-16.00hrs (Sat & Sun 12.00-16.00hrs subject to staff availability)

coffee shop

Situated on the first floor concourse and is open Mon-Fri 07.30-20.00hrs.

w.r.v.s. coffee bar

Situated on the ground floor opposite J&K Clinic is open Mon-Fri 9.30 - 5.00, Sat 12.30 - 4.00.

W.R.V.S. Coffee Bar
(Linda McCartney Centre)

Situated on the ground floor of the Linda McCartney Centre is open Mon-Fri 10.00 - 5.00

dining room

Situated on the lower ground floor is open

Mon-Sun	
0.7.30-11.00hrs	Breakfast
Closed	
12.00-14.00hrs	Lunch
14.30-15.30hrs	Closed
15.30-17.00hrs	Drinks/Snacks
17.00-20.00hrs	Evening Meal
20.00hrs	Closed
23.00-03.00hrs	Snacks & Drinks

mail box

Situated near the main Hospital entrance. Stamps are available from the League of friends shop.

autobank

Situated on the first floor concourse.

pay phone

Available on each floor outside the ward areas and in the main Hospital entrance.

Smoking

There is a strict No Smoking Policy throughout the Hospital with designated areas where you can smoke. Please discuss this with the ward staff.

Accommodation

As far as possible the ward staff will make a comfortable chair available at the bedside if you are staying with your loved one overnight. The ward staff will indicate the nearest toilet and washroom facilities for your use.

Hillsborough Suite

Accommodation is available close to the main Hospital complex, at a nominal charge, please ask ward staff if you would like more information.

Appendix 6

Bereavement leaflet

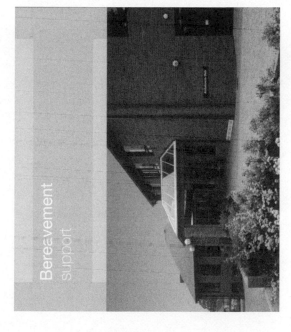

Bereavement support

Marie Curie
Cancer Care

1) LIVERPOOL BEREAVEMENT SERVICE
(formerly CRUSE)
25, Hope Street
LIVERPOOL L1 9PQ
Tel: 0151 - 708 6706

2) AGE CONCERN
2, Sir Thomas Street
LIVERPOOL L1
Tel: 0151 - 236 4440

3) MERSEYSIDE AIDS SUPPORT GROUP
Tel: 0151 - 708 9080

4) SAMARITANS
Tel: 0151 - 708 8888

5) BACUP
Freeline 0808 800 1234
Will give you details of bereavement support in your area.
www.cancerbacup.org.uk

6) COMPASSIONATE FRIENDS (Death of child regardless of age)
Helpline 0117 953 9639
www.tcf.org.uk

7) LESBIAN AND GAY BEREAVEMENT PROJECT
Helpline 020 8455 8894
www.members.aol.com/LGBP

Judith Williamson
Principal Social Worker

Marie Curie Centre Liverpool

The Marie Curie Centre Liverpool is one of ten Marie Curie Centres, providing specialist inpatient and outpatient care and day therapy. The Charity also runs research and education centres and a nursing service, enabling people to be cared for at home when this is their choice.

In the Centre, care is provided by highly skilled multi-professional health teams - doctors, nurses, social work, and welfare rights team, occupational and physiotherapists, spiritual/pastoral carers and complementary therapists. Our care provides relief from pain and other distressing symptoms, aiming to meet the physical, psychological, spiritual, cultural and social needs of patients and their family - helping make the most of life.

Marie Curie Centre Liverpool
Speke Road
Woolton
Liverpool L25 8QA
Tel: 0151 801 1400

Marie Curie Cancer Care
89 Albert Embankment
London SE1 7TP
Charity Reg No. 207994

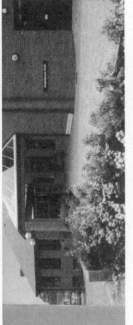

Bereavement
support

Bereavement is something which most people experience at some time in their lives, and people react to it in different ways. Grief, though painful, is not an illness and you need not be alarmed by the feelings and symptoms it sometimes causes. However, you may find the following information helpful.

It can be hard to accept the loss. You may experience a sense of shock and you may find yourself denying that the death has occurred. It is not unusual to think that you may have heard or seen the person who has died. In addition, many bereaved people feel strained and physically run down, finding it difficult to eat or sleep, and maybe feel tearful. Grief is time-consuming and exhausting.

You may find that you have lost all interest in living. Despair and depression may make you feel that there is no point in going on or that no-one else could possibly experience what you are going through. You may need reassurance that all these are natural reactions to bereavement and not a sign that you are 'going mad' or letting down your family and friends.

As well as feeling grieved and sad, you must also be prepared for any of the following: guilt, panic, self-pity and anger - even at the person who has died. If you do experience any of these emotions, you may feel you ought to hide them, but they too are part of grieving; don't be afraid to share them with a sympathetic listener. You may find yourself feeling hurt, convinced perhaps, that some of your family, friends or neighbours are avoiding you. Unfortunately, this often happens and is probably due to their embarrassment, not knowing what to say. It may be necessary for you to take the first step and let them know you would appreciate their support.

It is sometimes very tempting to feel that life would be more bearable if you moved house, or quickly disposed of possessions, or refused to see people. There is a very natural urge to avoid painful things. However, this usually makes things worse and decisions like these must be given careful thought. Bereavement is a time of very painful emotions which you will need to face and work through, before eventually beginning to rebuild your life.

With the passage of time, when the pain has eased a little, you will find yourself being able to remember without becoming so distressed. This can be a time for you to start taking up life afresh and it is important that you try to renew old interests and perhaps take up new pursuits. This might seem disloyal to the person who has died, but what has happened in the past is always a part of you and is not affected by your enjoying the present.

Grief is a very individual process and everyone reacts differently, so don't feel that you are in any way abnormal if yours does not appear to follow the pattern outlined here. It is important to allow yourself to grieve; but it is also important to take a break from grieving from time to time and eventually put it aside, even though you will never put aside the memories of the one you loved.

For those people whose relative or friend has died at the Marie Curie Centre, Liverpool, bereavement support is available. Social Workers, and trained volunteer bereavement visitors offer a follow-up service on a one-to-one basis. Bereavement Support Groups are also organised on a regular basis.

A Children and Young People's Counsellor is available for the younger members of the family who may also be finding this a difficult and confusing time.

If you would like details of these services or would like to talk to someone about your situation, please contact Judith Williamson, Principal Social Worker on 0151-801 1423 (direct line).

You may find it helpful to contact your local clergy or your G.P. Overleaf are details of other organisations that may also offer support, particularly if you live outside the Liverpool area.

Appendix 7

Symptom control guidelines

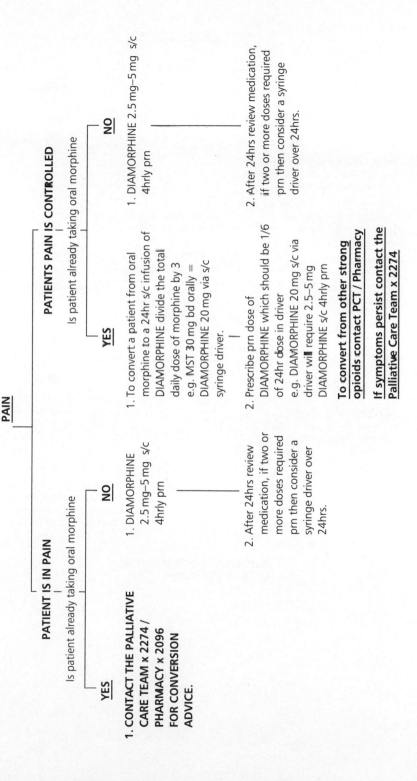

PAIN

PATIENT IS IN PAIN

Is patient already taking oral morphine

YES

1. CONTACT THE PALLIATIVE CARE TEAM x 2274 / PHARMACY x 2096 FOR CONVERSION ADVICE.

NO

1. DIAMORPHINE 2.5 mg–5 mg s/c 4hrly prn

2. After 24hrs review medication, if two or more doses required prn then consider a syringe driver over 24hrs.

PATIENTS PAIN IS CONTROLLED

Is patient already taking oral morphine

YES

1. To convert a patient from oral morphine to a 24hr s/c infusion of DIAMORPHINE divide the total daily dose of morphine by 3 e.g. MST 30 mg bd orally = DIAMORPHINE 20 mg via s/c syringe driver.

2. Prescribe prn dose of DIAMORPHINE which should be 1/6 of 24hr dose in driver e.g. DIAMORPHINE 20 mg s/c via driver will require 2.5–5 mg DIAMORPHINE s/c 4hrly prn

To convert from other strong opioids contact PCT / Pharmacy

If symptoms persist contact the Palliative Care Team x 2274

NO

1. DIAMORPHINE 2.5 mg–5 mg s/c 4hrly prn

2. After 24hrs review medication, if two or more doses required prn then consider a syringe driver over 24hrs.

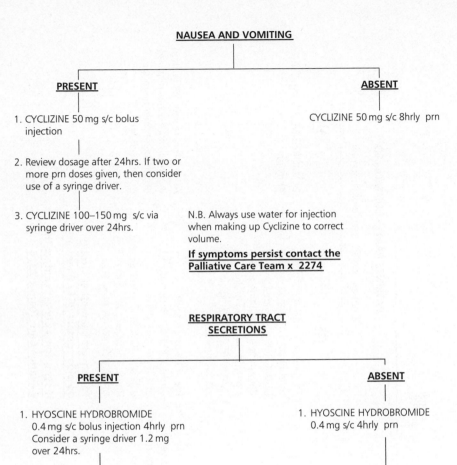

NAUSEA AND VOMITING

PRESENT

1. CYCLIZINE 50 mg s/c bolus
   injection

2. Review dosage after 24hrs. If two or
   more prn doses given, then consider
   use of a syringe driver.

3. CYCLIZINE 100–150 mg s/c via
   syringe driver over 24hrs.

ABSENT

CYCLIZINE 50 mg s/c 8hrly prn

N.B. Always use water for injection
when making up Cyclizine to correct
volume.
**If symptoms persist contact the
Palliative Care Team x 2274**

**RESPIRATORY TRACT
SECRETIONS**

PRESENT

1. HYOSCINE HYDROBROMIDE
   0.4 mg s/c bolus injection 4hrly prn
   Consider a syringe driver 1.2 mg
   over 24hrs.

2. Continue to give prn dosage
   accordingly.

3. Increase total 24hr dose to 2.4 mg
   after 24hrs if symptoms persist.

ABSENT

1. HYOSCINE HYDROBROMIDE
   0.4 mg s/c 4hrly prn

2. If two or more doses of prn
   HYOSCINE HYDROBROMIDE
   equired then consider a syringe
   driver s/c over 24hrs.

**If symptoms persist contact the
Palliative Care Team x 2274**

TERMINAL RESTLESSNESS
& AGITATION

PRESENT

1. MIDAZOLAM 2.5–5 mg s/c 4 hrly
   prn

2. Review the required medication after
   24hrs, if two or more prn doses have
   been required then consider a syringe
   driver over 24 hrs.

3. Continue to give prn dosage
   accordingly.

ABSENT

1. MIDAZOLAM 2.5–5 mg s/c 4 hrly
   prn

2. If two or more doses required prn,
   consider use of a syringe driver over
   24 hrs.

**If symptoms persist contact the
Palliative Care Team x 2274**

Index